Advance Praise

for *The 7 Principles of Health*

"Those looking for answers to health issues in both conventional and alternative medicine may find them in this remarkable book. In sharing her story, Natasha Deonarain, an M.D. who found answers to her own life-threatening illnesses, unites the art and science of medicine and shows us how we can do the same."
— Gladys Taylor McGarey, M.D. MD[H]

"A timely self-help book that encourages individuals to re-examine their health care. Deonarain, a family practitioner with several urgent-care clinics in Arizona, writes in this debut that doctors, including herself, are trained to "preach disease." To remedy this, she asserts, people need to take control of their health care choices, making themselves — not their health care provider or plan — the center of the decision-making process. Deonarain's own personal health history provides a great example of how a new health care perspective saved her life. An often engaging plan for taking control of one's health."
— *Kirkus Reviews*

"Dr. Deonarain provides a blueprint for empowerment that helps us see beyond the limitations and flaws of our disease-oriented conventional medical model. She teaches us to examine our attitudes toward illness and how to become active participants in the creation and practice of personal health. An important book for all who wish to take responsibility for their own healthcare decisions."
— LARRY MALERBA, DO, DHt, author of *Green Medicine: Challenging the Assumptions of Conventional Health Care*

Advance Praise

for *The 7 Principles of Health*

"*The 7 Principles of Health* is a real wake-up call. Finally we hear from a doctor who's not afraid to share what needs to change so we all can achieve optimal health, instead of just covering up the underlying issues with band-aids. This is a must read if you want to start taking control of your health and well-being."
— **Scott White, personal trainer, Personal Power Training**

"I could not put this book down. *The 7 Principles of Health* is unlike any book on health you have read. It is NOT about disease; it is about the power of our marvelous bodies to heal. All our talk about 'Health Care Reform'? THIS IS IT!"
— **Naomi Rhode, CSP, CPAE Speaker Hall of Fame/Past President National Speakers Association/Past President Global Speakers Federation/Cofounder, SmartHealth**

From my heart to yours,
natasha 2013

The
7 Principles
of Health™

From my heart to yours,
Natasha

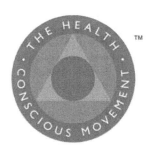

The 7 Principles *of* Health™

YOUR CALL TO HEALTH
CONSCIOUSNESS

Natasha N. Deonarain, MD, MBA

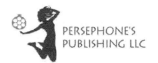

Copyright ©2013 Natasha Deonarain, M.D., MBA and Health Conscious Movement™
All rights reserved.
Printed in the United States of America.

Except as permitted under the United States Copyright Act of 1976, no part of this publication may be reproduced or distributed in any form or by any means, or stored in a database or retrieval system, without prior written consent of the publisher. Requests for permission or further information should be addressed to the Health Conscious Movement Permissions Department.

NOTE: This book is not intended as medical advice. The reader should consult his or her personal healthcare practitioner, particularly with respect to any symptoms that may require diagnosis or medical attention.

ISBN 978-0-988-60960-0

Health Conscious Movement
Health-Conscious.org

Cover and interior design by Bill Greaves, Concept West.

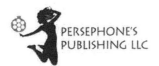

PERSEPHONE'S
PUBLISHING LLC

To you, with unconditional love —

sans commencement, sans fin.

TABLE OF CONTENTS

The
7 Principles
of Health™

CHAPTER ONE: Introduction 1

CHAPTER TWO: Overview of *The 7 Principles of Health* 26

CHAPTER THREE: Principle 1: Be Present 53

CHAPTER FOUR: Principle 2: Become Aware 71

CHAPTER FIVE: Principle 3: Be Health 98

CHAPTER SIX: Principle 4: Reawaken Curiosity 119

CHAPTER SEVEN: Principle 5: Channel Creativity 145

CHAPTER EIGHT: Principle 6: Grow and Renew 163

CHAPTER NINE: Principle 7: Heal, Change, and Thrive 190

CHAPTER TEN: Epilogue 204

ACKNOWLEDGMENTS 217

ABOUT THE AUTHOR 219

INDEX 221

The
7 Principles
of Health™

CHAPTER ONE

Introduction

"The first duties of the physician are
to educate the masses not to take medicine."

— **Sir William Osler** *(1849-1919)*
Canadian physician and professor of medicine

People tell me stories all the time. It's my job to listen.

Hope was 27 years old when she came into my office, depressed and overweight. She told me she couldn't shed a pound although she "ate like a bird." She found it difficult to concentrate at work, and her relationships with her husband and kids were becoming more stressful than ever. She was beginning to feel that something was terribly wrong, so she decided to visit her doctor.

"What did he do?" I asked.

"I told him my story," she said. "I was getting sore all over, I mean really sore, as though I'd been working out all the time. It was really weird. But when I did try to work out, even go for a walk, I couldn't. I was so exhausted, I couldn't believe it — like I could hardly lift my legs to take a step. So he ordered some blood tests and when they came back, he told me they were all normal."

"What did he advise?"

She laughed without humor. "He told me to diet and exercise. But you don't understand! I hardly eat, honestly. I've been trying to get an exercise program going, but I'm so tired all the time." She hesitated for a moment. "So he gave me a prescription for some pain medication."

"To treat what?"

"For my aches and pains."

"Did it help?"

"No. I felt even worse. So I went back to him and told him that something must be wrong. My hands and feet were beginning to swell."

"Then what happened?" I asked.

"He ran some more blood tests. They were all normal, too. So he gave me another pill, a water pill."

"Did that one work?" I prodded her to continue.

"Right," she said, her lip pinching tight. "He told me I probably had those symptoms because I wasn't exercising enough. And then he gave me a sleeping pill."

"What was that for?"

"To help me sleep," she replied, staring at me hard, as if she were questioning my professional competence.

"But what's the problem?" I asked.

"I don't know!" she exclaimed, throwing her hands up in frustration. "I was hoping you could tell me that."

"Did you see any other doctors?" I continued.

She rolled her eyes. "I went back to the same guy again. I've just been feeling awful and the pills weren't working. He just got really short with me, as if he was angry I had come back again. But I was desperate, Doctor."

"So what did he do this time?"

"He gave me a prescription for an antidepressant. Oh, and a referral to an endocrinologist."

"Why'd he do that?"

"Well, he said he wanted to make sure that there was nothing else wrong with my hormones, although my thyroid tests had come back normal. Oh yeah, and another referral — to a psychiatrist."

"What for?"

"He said I was depressed."

"What did those doctors do?"

"They repeated my blood tests," she replied, matter-of-factly. "The endocrinologist said I was fine. He made me feel like it was all in my head and told me that the antidepressant probably just needed more time to kick in. He told me to diet and exercise. The psychiatrist listened for a total of one minute and was already writing the prescription as I was telling him my story."

"What did he give you?"

"Another antidepressant," she sighed. "And a different sleeping pill. That one was way too expensive, so I didn't fill the prescription."

INTRODUCTION | 3

"Are they going to see you again?"

"No. They told me to go back to my primary care doc and lose more weight." She looked up at me. "But he's not helping me. I saw him again — I didn't want to but I had to. I think ... I think Jason's going to leave me." Her eyes welled with tears. "But I'm in pain all the time now, and nothing's working. I'm so tired all the time. I can't get up in the morning because I take the sleeping pill at night. It's a nightmare. It's like I want to sleep, but can't. I don't think I can do this anymore."

"What did your primary say when you went back to him?"

"He gave me a stronger pain pill. A narcotic. And he told me my cholesterol was high and that I was pre-diabetic. He told me again that I'd better diet and exercise or I was going to be diabetic soon and have to start taking medication. That's when he referred to me a cardiologist and a gynecologist."

"More specialists? Why?"

"Well, my heart." She gave me another hard look, as if it should have been obvious to a 2-year-old.

"What's wrong with your heart?" I asked.

"I don't know. The primary doc told me I should go see the heart doctor. And also the gynecologist."

"For a routine exam?"

"No. My periods have been really heavy and irregular. My gynecologist tried putting me on the pill, but it didn't work."

"So which pills are you currently taking?"

"Oh, God, I can't keep track. Cholesterol, sleeping, birth control, antidepressants — but I bought the cheaper one, the other one cost too much — the narcotic for pain, ibuprofen..." She listed each drug, tapping her fingers one by one. "I think something for blood pressure." Her eyes widened suddenly. "Did you know that cholesterol pill he prescribed costs $300 a month! I can't afford that."

"Did he have any other suggestions?"

She nodded. "He told me to diet and exercise."

●

It seems I've heard this same story, again and again. All I have to do is change the names. In every case, I get the sense that these patients are desperately searching for something they haven't been able to find.

4 | THE 7 PRINCIPLES OF HEALTH

Despite being told by doctors that there's nothing wrong, they know something is amiss. In each case, after drifting through the convoluted maze and confusion of a modern healthcare system that promises health, they end up sicker and more frustrated than ever.

Perhaps Hope's story is also your story.

What happened to bring us to this point? How did we get here? We spend nauseating amounts of money on our desperate search for health and healing, but we remain sick, tired, and broke. Lasting health and happiness in this amazing, high-tech medical system still seems to elude us.

The problem seems immense. In addition to the relationship breakdown between doctor and patient, and the increasingly adversarial relationship over money, prescriptions, wills, and wants, lays a paralysis. Doctors feel unable to heal their patients or their professions. Patients feel unable to find personal health and wellness.

These are some of the words we often hear tossed around: *fixes, cures, healthcare crisis, fragmented care, pills, fraud, blame, complaints, redundancy, lawsuit, victim, mandate, separate, individual, dictate, quack, lack of scientific evidence,* and *polarized care.* In America, we spend $2.5 trillion a year on healthcare, an amount that is projected to increase to $4.4 trillion by 2019[1]. We're paying more than ever before and we're all going broke. We're fragmenting our bodies and our social structure into the "haves" and the "have nots." Inside this mess, we're trying to get healthier, eat properly, diet and exercise, but instead of getting better, we keep getting worse and worse. We're frustrated. We seem to be caught in a paradoxical nightmare as we search for healing inside a system that operates to keep us sick. And we keep trying to fix it ourselves by doing the same things again and again.

Continuing down the same path in our personal search for health will not help us heal. Doing things the same old way inside our current medical system, as doctors and providers, will not solve our problems. We need a new way of thinking.

Hope's story is not unique. Her problems are the same ones many of us face or have faced within a system that's grossly out of control in its attempt to deliver health. Things have reached such a crisis that

---

[1]National Center for Health Statistics, United States, 2011: With Special Feature on Socioeconomic Status and Health. Hyattsville, MN. 2012

many of us may think we need more to solve these problems: more money, more healthcare services, more doctors, more resources, more technology, more cures — more of just about everything we feel we're lacking. We may think we'll never be able to get well because we simply can't afford it.

Is that the final answer, though? Or is it possible for you and I to find optimal health while paying less — much, much less than the sky-rocketing bills that we currently receive from hospitals, therapists, and doctor's offices? Is it possible to live a better life, one that's not consumed by disease-focused thinking at every turn we make inside our current healthcare system? It's no wonder we're struggling — the paradox we're facing has been carefully hidden from view. We have not been provided healthcare in America and in many Western countries. In fact, the exact opposite is true: we are actively prevented from finding health or accessing the ability to heal ourselves. It's simply impossible to do such things within a system that was created to keep us ill through fear, distraction and victimization. What we have created is *health-fear*. And this fear has disempowered us and turned us into victims who are willing to pay endless amounts of money for an unattainable promise: the promise of health.

> "We cannot solve our problems by using the same thinking we used when we created them."
>
> — Albert Einstein

The problem, quite simply, is our focus on disease. Whether or not we've been diagnosed with illness, we will never — either as individuals or as a collective society — be able to heal or find health by beginning with disease. Yet, it is this diseaseobsessed thinking that forms the basis of our healthcare system today. If we truly desire to break free and find optimal health, we must first change ourselves. And in order to change ourselves, we must first change the way we see things and the way we think.

●

The following is a letter I recently received from a patient.

Hi Natasha,

I'm wondering if you have any feedback or can provide me with a recommendation. I've had high blood pressure since my pregnancy

6 | THE 7 PRINCIPLES OF HEALTH

with my third daughter. It remained untreated and went up to 180/80 and has remained stubborn ever since. I've also had a pinhole tear in my aorta since 1980, which was repaired surgically. I was put on a fistful of medications, including several for my blood pressure, but it's still hard to control. I've been under good cardiac care for many years and followed up twice a year for regular checkups, blood work, echocardiograms, MRIs, and stress testing.

Recently, I started having rhythm problems and noticed an increase in my blood pressure, but I couldn't figure out what was causing it. I've had some added stress with going back to graduate school and trying to finish my degree. I had a nuclear stress test a few weeks ago which showed the possibility of a reversible defect or ischemia (lack of oxygen to the heart). Everything else was normal. My doctor said this might be something called an artefact or incidental finding. I've had no chest pain, shortness of breath, or any other problem and have not had any trouble exercising, but I've been strongly advised to avoid it. I had a recent echocardiogram that aroused no suspicion. I had a second one, but it seems, as per the stress test, the results are now unclear. There was also some confusion as to which medications I should take and which I should avoid.

In any case, my doctor recommended an angiogram and I was told to be prepared to stay overnight in case they had to fix something. While I recognize that this may be a necessity, further reading on my part has raised several questions, especially what will happen if this test indicates that other procedures might be needed. I'm afraid this is taking on a life of its own; it feels as though I'm running down a path to further and more invasive procedures without adequate time to investigate my options. I'm aware that there are other forms of diagnostic procedures which may be less invasive and would leave me less at the mercy of an interventional cardiologist whose incentive is to perform more tests and procedures whether I need them or not.

Part of my concern is that my doctor has folded his practice into a larger corporation and I have been VERY dissatisfied with the administrative aspects of my visits since his transition. It seems I no longer have ANY access to discuss issues with him outside of an office visit. I cancelled my scheduled appointment for the angiogram until I feel more comfortable about the whole thing.

INTRODUCTION | 7

I think I have other issues that haven't been considered or investigated and I would like to find someone who is more likely to take a broad view that includes ALL of my history. Please contact me at your earliest convenience.

Sincerely,

Sharon

This book offers a solution for people like Hope and Sharon — and you. It offers a new way of thinking about our personal health in the context of our current medical system. It will show us — both patients and doctors — that there is a new way to heal: simply by changing our paradigm.

Paradigms

The word *paradigm* is trendy these days. Many of us like to say we've *shifted our paradigm*, changed our perspective, or now practice "out-of-the-box" thinking. Paradigm can be defined as a way of looking at things. It is, essentially, a viewpoint comprised of a conglomeration of thoughts, also known as our mindset. Each of us is unique. My mindset or perspective may be similar to yours, but it is more than likely different in some way.

When we talk about changing perspectives, paradigms, or mindsets, the out-of-box concept is often used. But a friend of mine made this observation: "There are no boxes except the ones we've put ourselves inside." You've likely heard — or used — a few common phrases that demonstrate this concept of differing perspectives:

"The glass is half-empty."

"No, it's half-full."

"This is a crisis!"

"No, it's a great opportunity."

"Our society is better off than it was 50 years ago."

"No way — it's much worse!"

Your point of view is the way *you* see things. It is the paradigm or perspective from which you operate. When it comes to our personal health and healthcare system, we tend to view things through a common perspective. Many of us believe that the goal of our healthcare

8 | THE 7 PRINCIPLES OF HEALTH

system and its components (doctors, hospitals, health insurance companies, drug companies, and/or government health programs) is to make or keep us healthy. We think that doctors help us heal and that we pay health insurance companies to prevent us from getting sick or to help cover the cost of our fixes when we are broken and ill.

But what if I told you that the entire setup of our medical system — and the way we deliver healthcare — is designed to keep us sick, unhealthy, and financially broke? Would you believe me if I told you that from my perspective (as a physician who was trained inside the conventional medicine model), if you enter our medical system as a healthy person and see a doctor like myself for a "checkup," we doctors will turn your thoughts away from health and replace it with a disease-focused thinking. It's true. We'll preach disease, which will cause you to stress out about the possibility of contracting said illness. You'll act with the goal of preventing or fixing disease, rather than focusing on health first, regardless of whether any disease is even present. You'll focus so intently on disease thoughts that you will forget about health or what it means to practice health. You may still think you're healthy because you've had a checkup and you haven't been diagnosed with any disease. Generally, though, you'll become more concerned about disease within the context of healthcare, so much so that you'll turn all your thoughts, beliefs, and actions toward disease, cures, fixes, and prevention — rather than living healthy.

Do such statements shock you? This new and possibly controversial or contentious perspective may have stirred a reaction in you. Perhaps you don't agree with me. Perhaps you think I'm crazy, wonder what I'm up to, or think it's heresy to hear a doctor saying that the medical system has been set up to cause disease.

Let's return to our discussion on paradigms for just a moment. This particular observation is my perspective, my way of seeing things, and not necessarily yours. So who is right? Is your perspective reality, or is my perspective reality? How do we know what's reality when it comes to health and healthcare? Is there only one perspective we should all share? Could the perspective we've clung to for so long simply be a point of view conferred on us by others? Sometimes the boxes we build for ourselves have very thick walls.

Try for a moment to see my perspective. Could my way of seeing things lead you to change the way you think about healthcare? Could my perspective prompt you to give more thought to your ability to find optimal health and longevity? Is it possible that by changing your perspective, you could create a new starting point that would take you on a very different journey to health than the path you're currently following? Might you begin to see a different paradigm emerging from the one that's been so well entrenched in our society?

We all know by now that we are sick, as individuals and as a nation. Just look at the latest headlines and read a few sobering health statistics and you'll know it's true. Isn't it safe to say that healthcare as we see it isn't really healthcare? From my perspective, it certainly doesn't seem to be doing what it's supposed to do, which is care for our health.

When it comes to paradigms, Stephen Covey, author of *The 7 Habits of Highly Effective People*, has this to say:

> While individuals may look at their own lives and interactions in terms of paradigms or maps emerging out of their experience and conditioning, these maps are not the territory. They are a "subjective reality," only an attempt to describe the territory.

Is it possible we were given the wrong map to follow on our journey to find and maintain our health?

The "reality" of our medical system is purely subjective. It was constructed from our collective perspective, and under its construct, we have been taught to believe in it — unquestioningly. This belief in traditional medicine has become so ingrained that we're having trouble realizing we're all stuffed inside a very deep box. The healthcare stakeholders' primary interest is having us continue to believe that our medical system must be the way it is today. What we've failed to realize, however, from our perspective deep within our box, is that their motive differs vastly from ours. They are hell-bent on making sure we see only one view of how healthcare should be delivered. For too long now, doctors and patients — you and I — have all tacitly agreed to believe this singular perspective.

The thing about our box is that it doesn't exist unless we believe it exists. So if we're all going to find real, lasting health and learn how to heal ourselves — individually and collectively — we're going to

10 | THE 7 PRINCIPLES OF HEALTH

have to consider changing our way of thinking first. We must agree to dismantle our deceptive box.

Principles

What are principles? Principles are natural laws that cannot be broken. Dan Millman, in his Warrior Athlete book series, states that these laws are "sewn into the fabric of existence."

Generally, we can define a principle as "a general truth or law, basic to other truths."[2] When it comes to our health, there are certain principles that cannot be broken. Let's say we decide to eat an unrestricted diet of high-fructose corn syrup, saturated fat, and processed food. We then choose to sit on our couch and watch television for four hours or more a day. What principle have we violated in this example?

Everything in life is in balance. From darkness to light, day to night, birth to death, creation to destruction — our world and everything in it is in total balance. This includes us and our health. By eating an excess of unhealthy foods and avoiding exercise, we have violated the principle or law of balance. We cannot escape this fundamental truth and expect to be healthy.

The 7 Principles of Health are laws that are woven into our human spirit. They are part of our being. If we align ourselves with these principles, we can reawaken our own innate ability to heal. Dan Millman goes on to say that "when we align our lives — our habits of diet, exercise, work, and sexuality — with spiritual laws, challenges remain, but we can approach them without struggle, with arms open wide, like peaceful warriors embracing the moment, ready to dance." *The 7 Principles of Health* can help us realign ourselves to optimal health. They represent a new roadmap to our desired destination. They replace the original map we received and which we have, unfortunately, been following far too long.

Let's use an example to illustrate this point. Say you want to travel from Phoenix to L.A. If someone gave you a map from New York to Boston to follow, you might eventually reach your destination, but with no help from the map. In the context of our current healthcare system and the health paradigm within which we function, *The 7*

---

[2]*Funk and Wagnalls Standard Desk Dictionary*, Harper & Row, Publishers, Inc. 1984

Principles of Health are a new guide to help us reach our destination: optimal health.

Practices

In this book, I also outline *The 5 Disciplines of Health Practice*™. Practices are habits. These are the actions we do every day, or on most days, which hardly enter our conscious mind. They are not necessarily glamorous or exciting, and in fact may be quite boring to some. But they are the actions we carry out in our day-to-day lives which must be in alignment with our guiding principles.

When it comes to personal health, we often hear words like: *diet and exercise, take these pills, lose weight,* and *control your blood pressure.* These are not habits. These are simply items on a list of commands that often come from someone else, namely someone like me, a doctor. To develop healthful practices, we must go deeper and choose those actions that align with our principles, which means they may not necessarily agree with the commands we receive from our doctors.

Of course, habits and practices can be constructive or destructive. As we pursue health, we must realize that our habits or acts can maximize or destroy our health. The choice is ours to make. If optimal health is our goal, it will be important to develop constructive practices to lead us there. We may not always execute them perfectly, but we simply cannot escape from the practices or habits we keep on a daily basis. They will, in every instance, determine our outcomes.

Requirements

If you were to ask someone you know to travel with you to Alaska, what would be some of the requirements of your friend? In addition to money, time, etc., your friend would also need one fundamental requirement: the desire to go. Say he or she said they really didn't want to go unless you threatened them (and hopefully you wouldn't!). If they agreed to take the trip anyway, it would probably be because they still had some unspoken desire to go. They'd want to hang out with you, they'd really want to go to Alaska, or both.

Similarly, ask someone to get healthy. Ask them to diet and exercise, eat more fiber, monitor their blood sugar, or reduce the amount

12 | THE 7 PRINCIPLES OF HEALTH

of stress in their life. They wouldn't do it unless they had the desire to change. The desire to change ourselves for the sake of attaining better health is an example of an attitude we must have individually in order to achieve health. We must want to be healthy, not just to run away from disease. We can try and force people to change by increasing the amount they pay for insurance, by getting angry, or by punishing them if they don't have health insurance. We can force doctors to pay if their

> *"The way in which we see the problem is the problem."*
>
> — Stephen Covey

patients don't get healthy. But until an individual patient truly wants to change, no one will be able to make them do so.

So, underlying *The 5 Disciplines of Health Practice* are *The 7 Requirements for Health Practice.* These are attitudes and steps each of us must honor in order to find optimal health.

The Problem

What is our actual healthcare problem? Let's take a closer look at how we see our current health system. Here are some examples of words and phrases we use to describe our current situation in medicine. I've added more information next to the key words to help explain some of them.

Current Health Paradigm

Quick Fix	Rapid cures, band-aid solutions, band-aid cures
Fragmentation	Broken apart, disjointed, disconnected, unconnected, redundant, separated into pieces or subcomponents
Individualism	Concerned with the person as individual vs. the common, group, or collective interest; egoism; placing priority on individuals first, and not the collective; lack of sharing; concern with the self over others; prioritizing "me" first

Cure	Eliminate, correct, restore, get rid of, fix
Disease Orientation	Focusing on a disordered or non-functioning part, structure, or system; targeting study, prevention, and cure toward the abnormal or sickened component of the human body
Mechanization	Separating the whole into its interrelated parts; Newtonian physics; mechanistic; the sum of a body's parts equates to the whole when put together; focusing on individual parts instead of complex, integrated systems; using cause and effect instead of integrated functions
Polarization	At opposite ends of the spectrum; separated or divided; apart (EXAMPLES: conventional vs. complementary/alternative; East vs. West; allopathic vs. holistic; traditional vs. natural medicine)
Victimization	Disempowerment; lack of choice; doing things as you've been told; having things done to you against your will; lack of will power
Paternalism	Parent/child relationship comprised of orders, rules, dictates, management, or governance with punishment and/or reward; physician/doctor-centered models in medicine
Mandates	Dictates; orders; being told what to do; punishment as a consequence; bureaucracy; outside party involvement; command or demand to act in a particular way
Blame	To hold someone else responsible; lack of responsibility or accountability; to find fault in someone or something else
Judgment	Determination; conclusion; authoritative opinion; assessment or decision
Myopic Perspective	Narrow-sighted; tunnel-visioned; near-sighted; close-minded; narrow-minded; small picture view vs. big picture view; short-sighted
Unconsciousness	Unaware; not perceived at the level of awareness; not brought into one's conscious mindset or thinking

14 | THE 7 PRINCIPLES OF HEALTH

What do you think of these words? Do you agree or disagree with some of them as they relate to your personal health or the American healthcare system? Many of these words can be used to describe the status quo in today's healthcare. These words are used by doctors, other professionals, and many health industry experts. Some of them are now carefully being used by the media and by politicians who have been forced to confront certain realities of the immense problems embedded in our society today.

Can you imagine a different table we could create, one that uses different words to describe a new perspective or paradigm in healthcare?

New Health Paradigm

Long Term	Longevity (as in long life); for a long period of time; long-lasting; far-reaching; for the longest time possible; for life or lifelong
Whole	Undivided; integrated; all parts connected; together; collective; entire person; integral; unbroken; intact; complete
Collective	Forming a whole; combined; characteristics of a group of individuals taken together (as in society); synergistic; concerned with the group instead of the individual; functioning as a unit as opposed to separate pieces; a sum of parts
Healing	Bring to optimal health; make functional again; to restore to completeness or become whole again
Health	A general condition of the whole; a focus on achieving optimal wellness or optimal function in many aspects of life (EXAMPLES: mental, emotional, physical, social, environmental, financial, etc.); relieving the presence of dis-ease (lack of ease); assisting the body to rid itself of disease and return to a state of vigor, energy, or vitality
Energetic System	Multidimensional; Einsteinian physics; integration; inseparability; quantum theories; the whole is more than the sum of its parts; a way of viewing things as complex systems, rather than mechanical parts; viewing things as integrated functions rather than separable parts

Balance	Bringing together opposing sides equally; giving equal weight to different sides; a state of equilibrium; adjusting the portions symmetrically; avoiding excesses of one thing; moderation
Empowerment	Giving power; choice; authority; operating by personal will; enablement; will power; self-authority; making your own decisions; having the will or authority to decide
Guide or Teacher	Teacher/student relationships; assist in another's decision making; help, accompany; provide knowledge; instruct; lead; collaborate; work together; share
Collaboration	Supporting or working with one another; cooperation; working together; give and take; shared-decision making
Accountability	Responsibility; holding the self responsible; obligation to oneself; self-drive; answerability to the self
Nonjudgment	Without critical assessment or opinion; objective; without criticizing; without inference; without critical opinion
Clear Vision	Seeing things clearly, as in perception; 20/20; state of being transparent; freedom from indistinctness or ambiguity
Consciousness	State of awareness; knowing; being aware; participating in all sensations, perceptions, or activities; full presence

What do you think of these new words? Do they represent our current way of viewing healthcare? Could they represent a new paradigm that health industry experts, politicians, doctors, and patients might want? Is it possible for you to see these words used within a new health delivery system in which you participate?

Which table seems to best fit the context of your personal search for greater health? Do you notice a difference between the first table, The Current Health Paradigm, and the second one, The New Health Paradigm?

Many of these words are used to describe the way we would like to envision our health and medical systems, especially these days as we continue to embroil ourselves in the worst healthcare crisis our nation has ever faced. They do represent a new way of looking at things — a new paradigm. And it might truly be possible for them to characterize a new type of healthcare model or a health system in which we could all participate.

We've agreed that just about all of us are struggling to get healthier these days. But unless we shift our words, our thoughts, and our focus, our struggles will continue against a backdrop of skyrocketing insurance costs, modern epidemics of illness, and extreme stress over our healthcare crisis. We are sick physically, mentally, emotionally, financially, and spiritually. It's no wonder we're succumbing to disease faster than any previous generation did. Now it's up to us to find our way back to health.

Revisit the words used in The New Health Paradigm. Do you think it might be possible for Hope or Sharon from the earlier stories to find lasting health by starting with a different viewpoint? What if they were to begin with words like *health, healing, integrated, whole person,* and *empowered,* instead of words like *disease, cure, quick fix,* and *short-sighted?* What if they used their personal willpower and self-accountability to choose their own path to health instead of being at the mercy of doctors and a healthcare system that's "taking on a life of its own," as Sharon writes?

In the next section, we'll explore this concept a little further.

A Paradigm Shift

What constitutes a paradigm shift? As an example, try reading the following statements aloud:

1. The Earth is flat.

2. The Earth is round.

What are your thoughts or reactions to these statements? Just about everyone now understands and believes that the Earth is round. Although we may not have seen it with our own eyes from space, we can rely on pictures and stories from others who have.

It wasn't until 1837 that the last of the geocentrists (people who believed the Sun and planets revolved around the Earth) decided there was enough evidence to believe Copernicus, who discovered that the Earth actually revolves around the Sun. Similarly, Sir Isaac Newton's physics explained our world in terms of mechanical parts, making us the observers. We simply had to take things apart and study them separately in order to understand them. Then Albert Einstein came along, theorizing that we are not separable from our world as observers, but instead we're integrated with it. Phenomena can therefore be viewed in terms of energy and systems which cannot be separated from the whole.

Now, try reading these two sentences aloud. Study your own reactions or thoughts.

1. Medicine treats disease.

2. Health reverses disease.

How do you feel about these statements? Do you agree more with one than the other? What about these next two sentences? What are your thoughts or reactions to these?

1. The Sun revolves around the Earth.

2. The Earth revolves around the Sun.

Contrast the above statements with the following:

1. The doctor is the center of medicine.

2. You are the center of your health.

Our modern world has moved on with its understanding of physics and its knowledge of the cosmos. Sadly, medical practice is still stuck in Newtonian theory which believes that we can break our human bodies apart to be studied and then put them back together for a cure or a fix. How long will it take for us to stop modeling the geocentrists and understand that we need a new paradigm from which to operate?

Consider these next two statements and examine your reactions or thoughts.

1. Humans (we) are separate from the Universe.

2. Humans (we) are integrated with our Universe.

18 | THE 7 PRINCIPLES OF HEALTH

Now compare the following with what you the statements above:

1. I must be cured from disease (separated).

2. My body has an innate capacity to heal (integrated).

What do you think will happen if we don't change our mindset about health and medical practice? To answer this question, I think we have to look to the astronomers. In his book *Pale Blue Dot*, Carl Sagan takes us on a journey into space to explore our solar system and all that exists beyond it. He tells us that the space probes we've sent out to look for signs of life have found nothing. He tells us that it's a cold, dark, lonely universe, and that we haven't found any sign of other life for thousands of trillions of miles.

Sagan then shows us what Earth looks like from way up there. It turns out we're a miniscule pale blue dot that vanishes among a bunch of stars, asteroids, gas clouds, and other planets. He says that this blue dot we call Earth is the only home we have and he warns that we humans seem to be systematically destroying it.

Let's extrapolate from Sagan's premise: our bodies are the only homes we have, yet we seem to be quite comfortably destroying the sources of life that nourish our bodies: the air we breathe, the water we drink, and the foods we eat. We fail to understand that this earth, of which we are an integral part, is the source of everything we need to stay alive, never mind finding health. And at this juncture in our human existence, we've allowed ourselves to survive within the framework of a healthcare system that keeps us from seeing the big picture. And it is under this dark veil that we are systematically destroying our bodies, the only home we have.

The power of a paradigm shift can help us dramatically change this downward spiral. It can help us refocus as individuals and find personal health, happiness, and longevity. It can help us come together as a collection of people to create profound change in the way we perceive health and the way healthcare is delivered to us. It can help us change as a global community to construct a positive future for our children and grandchildren.

When we care about our only personal physical home, we cannot help but care about our only planetary home, the pale blue dot we call Earth. It's up to us to come together to figure this out, because we're it — there's no one else out there to help us.

A New Map

If we've been using the wrong map to find health for so long, how will we make a new one? How can we create a New Health Paradigm within this present situation that is so focused on illness and quick cures?

Stephen Covey says that everything we create has been created twice. In order to shift our paradigm and see something new, we must first create it in our minds. In order to create it in our minds, we have to learn to think differently. Let's take a look at how we can change our thoughts and thought forms. This is reprogramming our thoughts and our reactions to the way we think.

Thoughts and Thought Forms

Though they are invisible, our thoughts are essential to our progress as humans. Unlike this book (or eReader), these incomprehensible sparks of electrical energy in our brains are intangible. They cannot be seen, touched, or smelled, so how can they possibly produce something real, like a tumor in our bodies? How can thoughts bring into physical existence their very substance just by the mere fact that we're focusing on them?

You've probably heard about the power of positive thinking. But did you know that the reverse also is true? There's also such a thing as the power of negative thinking. Thoughts are very powerful. Whether positive or negative, thoughts can manifest outcomes or events in our lives. Maybe you've experienced this kind of cause and effect. When you think negatively, somehow negative things show up in your life. And conversely, when you think positively, your situations seem vastly different.

The fact is that an outcome or event is neither positive nor negative. It's our thinking that allows us to perceive a result as positive or negative in our minds. So the positivity or negativity of each event, circumstance, or occurrence depends solely on the person experiencing it and whether they consider the outcome to be a good or bad thing.

Recent work on neurolinguistic programming — changing our thought forms and perspectives — has the power to manifest change in our lives, including changes in our bodies, minds, and spirits. If we fill our minds with positive thoughts, goals, and intentions (health, for example), we can remap our brains to orient toward health. Our intentions are then carried out in the acts we perform every day; in this case, these acts are consistent with health. We begin paying attention to what we're eating every day, as opposed to going on a diet. We become aware of the kinds of food that nourish our bodies and the kinds of food that are toxic. We know which activities make us feel great and help us stay fit and healthy. We don't need doctors, our healthcare system, or the government to *tell* us what to do. We have access to all the information we need to become healthy; deep down inside, we know it's just common sense.

When we believe we are something, we are that thing: capable, happy, productive, and healthy. Likewise, when we believe we are not, we are not. It's as simple as that. So if we believe we are diseased, then worry about contracting a disease or getting sicker, and ultimately take actions to fight disease instead of practicing health, we paradoxically become the disease we most fear because we've programmed all of our thoughts, beliefs, and actions toward fighting it. We have not programmed them to health *first*. When our starting point is the belief that we are health, we naturally seek the professional health guides who are most knowledgeable about health practice, not disease practice. We learn how to carry out actions in our daily lives that promote optimal health, vitality, and vigor. As a result, we become healthy.

Disease-Oriented Thoughts

Why is our healthcare system so focused on disease? Let's take a closer look at how this came about.

The International Classification of Diseases (ICD) codes were formulated in the late 18th century as a compilation of statistics. The first comprehensive treatise on disease classification, Nosologia Methodica, was published by François Bossier de Lacroix (1706-1777). The classification system then evolved under Jacques Bertillion (1851-1922), who was Chief of Statistical Services of the city of Paris at the time. In 1898, The American Public Health Association adopted this system into North America (Mexico, Canada, and the United States), and since then, after ten revisions, it has become the ICD-10 codes. These disease codes constitute the skeleton of our medical system

INTRODUCTION | 21

today. The original list of about 100 causes of death has grown into hundreds of thousands.

How does this classification system affect us? Doctors use these codes to diagnose, primarily because they have been trained to find and focus on disease. They get paid to focus on disease. The numbers you see on your insurance bills are disease codes. Of these thousands of codes, very few are wellness or health codes, and those wellness codes are often ignored by doctors. The reason for this is very simple: doctors won't receive payments from the health insurance companies if you are found to be too healthy. The healthcare system and health insurance companies pay doctors to diagnose, treat, fix, and cure disease.

Let's say, for example, you're healthy. So you go into your doctor's office for a checkup, as confirmation. Your doctor sends you for a bunch of tests to screen for disease. Are you seeing the irony? He is looking for disease to determine whether you are healthy. He doesn't intend to find disease and really does want you to be healthy, but he's been trained to search for, find, and destroy disease. And further, unless he finds it, he won't get paid by the health insurance company that's told him he must find an illness in order to get paid.

And so, more likely than not, your doctor will find an illness of some sort to diagnose, and he may send you home with a bag full of pills or a list of tests to be performed. The thing is, it's not that hard to find something wrong with you these days. If you've got nothing *physical* wrong with you, you're probably stressed and anxious about healthcare and how you're going to pay for disease if you should get sick, about the future of our country, about the world you're leaving behind for your kids or your relatives' kids, or perhaps about your job. That stressed out condition is ICD-10 Code 308.0: *Stress Reaction, Emotional*. Making this diagnosis, as opposed to making no diagnosis at all (or, better still, a diagnosis of health), means your doctor can submit your bill and receive some sort of payment from your health insurance company.

Please understand, your doctor is not lying about your medical condition. This is just the way doctors must act under the framework of our present healthcare system. And this framework affects all of us. Health insurance companies do not pay doctors for health practice. They only pay doctors to fix, cure, and treat disease. Health insurance companies, and subsequently the doctors who must operate under them, find no wealth in keeping you healthy, so they make sure you're

22 | THE 7 PRINCIPLES OF HEALTH

afraid to get sick. They perpetuate the fear that you'll get sicker if you don't have health insurance. If you were less afraid of getting sick because you redirected the money you're now paying to insurance premiums to take good care of yourself by buying healthful foods and gym memberships, would you still be willing to pay these insurance companies tens of thousands of dollars each year?

Hospitals use the ICD system. Medicare uses the ICD system. Health insurance companies, lawyers, and the World Health Organization use the ICD system. Everyone associated with medicine in Western countries uses the ICD system. And we have taught you, as the patient, to understand the ICD system. We have taught you to focus your thoughts on disease and to fear death, rather than help you to focus first on finding optimal health. We have taught you to focus on eliminating disease first, and to search endlessly for a cure that's never going to be found. We have taught you to believe that only if you do not have a disease are you healthy.

Medicine creates disease. We give people pills or synthetic drugs that help certain symptoms of some diseases, but which also have the potential to create other problems. We then remove these synthetic pills from the market after they've harmed many people who initially thought they were safe. The cycle follows this pattern: doctors prescribe pills that are beneficial, until proven otherwise, to help us get healthy. These pills then often create new diseases or problems of which doctors initially were unaware. So the doctors slap disease labels on these new problems, making way for the creation of more pills and cures to address the new problems. The "new" diseases are added to the growing list of ICD codes. As we've mentioned, there are hundreds of thousands of diseases coded in the new ICD-10 classification system.

That's how it works. More pills are developed to counteract the diseases we created by prescribing pills in the first place. As you can see, our healthcare system and its conventionally trained doctors who have kept their focus trained on disease-focused thinking and practice actually create more and more disease, under the misguided belief that they are delivering health! Most conventionally trained doctors have never stopped to consider the big picture and the impact their part in the whole has had on patients and their own careers. It's a hidden

INTRODUCTION | 23

paradox that's perpetuated under the construct of modern healthcare and the way it is delivered to you.

Some doctors believe that naturopaths, acupuncturists, and chiropractors are nothing more than quacks who cannot help you find health. They discredit Eastern medical practices such as Traditional Chinese Medicine (TCM) or the use of herbs, stating that there is no scientific evidence to back up their efficacy or use. They don't want you to see alternative or holistic practitioners. One elderly colleague of mine recently called our acupuncturist a "voodoo medicine practitioner," despite the modality's growing popularity with patients.

Lawyers encourage you to sue doctors for malpractice. They advise you to focus on a particular disease and dig around to determine whether the doctor made a mistake by not curing or fixing you. They don't focus on your overall health. Lawyers don't get paid unless they convince you to blame someone for your ills, perpetuating your status as a victim of disease.

Our entire medical system is entrenched in disease-focused thought, and we have been sickened physically by this collective belief. This is a form of programming a particular belief system into our collective mindset, and the ubiquitous focus on disease represents the messages with which we are bombarded every day. We have as a society, collectively trained our brains to focus on disease, as opposed to health. No wonder we cannot easily find health inside our current healthcare system set-up. We're all using a disease-oriented map.

●

Allison is a friend of mine. She told me she'd been diagnosed with metastatic breast cancer. Her doctor informed her she had about 27 spots of cancer all over her bones, and that her liver and lungs also had cancer spots. The doctor also told her that she had perhaps two months to live.

That was five years ago.

"What did you do?" I asked her. "How did you go home with this diagnosis and prognosis — and live?!"

"It was so hard. It was unbelievable. Not only did I have to go home knowing that I was dying, but I was dropped by my insurance carrier. I lost my job and tried to get rehired, but no one wanted to hire someone like me. Employers realized that I'd cost them an arm and a leg in company health insurance."

"What happened?"

"I figured I had nothing left to lose. I had no insurance, no job, and pretty soon I wouldn't have a life. So you know what? I decided to live! I told myself that it was life or death, and I chose life. After all, what else did I have to lose?" She laughed jovially. Allison is vigorous, energetic, and absolutely glowing. "And look at me! I'm still alive! Even though they all tried to shit-can me!"

●

How can we shift our own personal paradigm enough so as to reorient our compass toward health instead of disease? You and I stand at the roots of change for our personal health. But if we're to succeed, we must also understand that we're intimately interconnected with our medical system and its collective thought environment. If the system is sick, we will all remain sick. If we each become healthy, the system will become healthy. The following diagram represents our relationship as individuals inside this medical system.

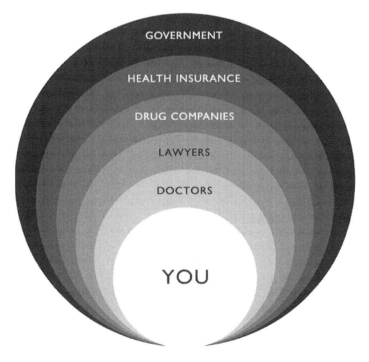

What's the solution to finding optimal health when our messaging system is primarily about disease? We can wait for outside parties to change our messages for us, such as health insurance companies, drug companies, lawyers, politicians, big corporations, or even doctors trained in this paradigm of disease. Or, we can take control of our own health and lives, deciding to change ourselves first.

To become health is to start from health. To begin with health, we must first see health and begin to practice it. In order

> *"For every 1,000 hacking at the leaves of evil, there is one striking at the root."*
>
> — **Henry David Thoreau**

to practice health, we must first change our paradigm. We must re-program our minds toward health in every moment and create new habits for ourselves. We must remove the deep boxes into which we have put ourselves and stand up against those messages that fight to pull us back toward disease. The *Health Conscious Movement*™ is designed to do just that.

This is your call to health consciousness. It's time to understand that you have only one home, and you must take care of it. By first beginning from health and seeking to practice it every moment of every day, you can create health in yourself and, as a result, in our healthcare system. You can become health conscious. You can then re-program your brain to think and carry out actions that are in alignment with health practice. And it will be this health practice — not medical practice — that will manifest optimal wellness in your life and correct many disease states. At this point in our history, shifting our paradigm has literally become a matter of life or death for every one of us.

Which will you ultimately choose?

CHAPTER TWO

Overview of
The 7 Principles *of* Health

"Natural forces within us are the true healers of disease."

— **Hippocrates** *(c 460 BC - c 370 BC)*
Ancient Greek physician, author of the Hippocratic Oath

The goal of the *Health Conscious Movement* is to fundamentally change our approach to health. When we change our paradigm to begin with health, rather than starting with disease, we are able to focus on all aspects of health in our lives. We can then stop practicing medicine, as doctors, patients, and institutions, and begin practicing health instead.

In order to do this, we must first understand the meaning of the word "health." It may sound basic, but in Western medical systems, we have interpreted this word to mean the absence of disease. But health is not merely the absence of disease. It is much more than that. Let's explore this concept a little further.

Health is a composite of our habits, which are born from our thought patterns or the messages we believe in. As we have mentioned, the messages we believe are referred to as programs, or scripts that make up our thought environment. The map or point of view from which we develop our habits or practices reflects our paradigm. We want to be sure that we're using the right map. With the proper map, we can act accordingly and find what we are looking for. So if we are looking for health, it makes sense that we begin with a health map or health perspective. But if we think, believe, and act in ways that focus on disease, disability, or sickness, we will become exactly that which we have programmed ourselves to think: diseased, disabled, and sick, no matter if we intended to find health in the first place. Conversely, if we think, believe, and act in ways that focus on health first, no matter what our *labels* of disease or disability might reflect, we become exactly what we think we are: healthy. We then think, act and live in total health. As we have seen with my friend Allison who was diagnosed with metastatic breast cancer, she began with her *belief* in health first. Then, she practiced health every day, turning her thoughts and actions into those that centered on health, not just the prevention of disease. It didn't matter which disease labels her doctor gave her, she focused on the big picture of optimal health. And by doing so, she outlived her own doctor's prognosis by many years!

The 7 Principles of Health are about learning how to begin a practice of health and how to stop practicing disease. That's not an easy thing to do in today's society and inside the messaging we constantly receive. Both doctors and patients are bombarded from many different sides, all of which reflect a message of disease. I believe this has formulated the basis for an increasingly adversarial relationship between doctors and their patients, propagated by external parties telling us which map to use, as you will come to discover in the course of this book. The consequence of not using the right map and the correct thought system or script comes with a steep price — for both parties. While we're trying to free ourselves from paying this steep price with our health and our personal finances, those external parties want to keep us enclosed inside a disease cage. In order to effect lasting change, we must find a new guide to use, a guide that will teach us how to heal.

How to Use This Book

As you read through the rest of these pages, you will encounter a tremendous amount of information. Some of it may seem overwhelming. When it comes to trying to understand the immense complexity of our current medical paradigm and the boxes we've all managed to put ourselves inside, the task before us may seem daunting.

The best way to learn new things is simply to begin with an open mind. It's not necessary to do anything just yet. Sit back, relax, and savor these sentences as if you were tasting a delicious meal. Do your best to refrain from any judgments about the information presented. Simply take the role of the observer for now. Allow the material of

28 | THE 7 PRINCIPLES OF HEALTH

The 7 Principles of Health to soak into you. Acknowledge any opinions you may hear yourself formulate as you read. Write down those thoughts, and then put them aside. Accept that they are your opinions and thoughts, but they are not necessarily right or wrong. You will likely find it very difficult to understand some of this information if you instantly respond from your old message system or well worn, preprogrammed thinking habits. Listening to that sort of input will only serve to create roadblocks on your journey to finding a new way of looking at things.

> *"Life is not measured by the breaths we take, but by the moments that take your breath away."*
>
> — **Hillary Cooper**

As you work your way through the material, you will have a chance to practice health with a few simple exercises, located at certain places within each chapter. Try them out, even if you take only a moment to think about them. It's important that you do the exercises. Try not to skip over them. They will help you process these new ideas in a very digestible format, and my hope is that by the end of the book, you'll be stimulated with the urge to learn more for yourself.

Once you've completed the book, the choice will then be yours. You may choose to reread the information and implement into your life, one principle at a time. My advice is to integrate small changes for at least 30 to 40 days. Don't try to do it all at once. Change takes time and is often a one-step-forward, two-steps-backward process. Going slowly and acting very deliberately, aware of what you're doing in each moment, will help you create habits or practices that last a lifetime.

You might choose to use my accompanying *The 7 Principles of Health Daily Progress Tracker* to help you keep track of the changes and progress you are making on a daily basis. This can be immensely useful for those tough days when you feel like you aren't getting anywhere and wonder to yourself, "How can ONE healthy meal really matter?" After just a few days of recording your progress, you'll begin to have measurable success to look back on so that you can stay motivated to make and meet new goals.

Finally, like any exciting adventure, you'll want to enjoy every moment. Don't rush through the material the same way we often rush through the moments of our lives. As you will come to see, failing to

OVERVIEW OF THE 7 PRINCIPLES OF HEALTH | 29

slow down and be present inside these wonderful episodes we call life is what has caused us all to become very sick. Our goal is to find a way to stop getting sicker and instead become healthy. So smile to yourself, curl up in a quiet place with your favorite drink, avoid any outside distractions (even for 15 minutes), and let's first take a look at the big picture.

The 7 Principles of Health

We'll begin with the following diagram. This is a representation of *The 7 Principles of Health* and the suggested direction in which you can proceed to learn each principle. I will refer back to it throughout the book.

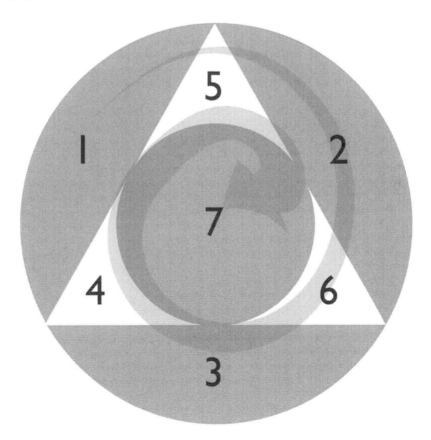

30 | THE 7 PRINCIPLES OF HEALTH

As you can see, *The 7 Principles of Health* are represented by a large circle with a triangle inside, and then another circle at the center. Principle 1 is represented on the top left section of the circle, dissected by one side of the triangle. As we continue learning about the different health principles, we will move from left to right, around the circle, continuing in a spiral. We then enter each corner section of the triangle and end inside the central circle, the heart of the entire shape.

Each of the different health principles is more easily understood by separating it from the others. In addition, each is best first experienced in the sequence presented, as you will come to understand. However, once you master each principle via the individual requirements and practices that underlie them, you'll discover that you can simultaneously and continuously practice all of *The 7 Principles* at once. They will become part of your being. They will come to represent who you are and, with that, your ability to find health. Are you ready to get started?

PRINCIPLE 1: Be Present

The first principle advises us to become centered. What does this mean? In today's highly distractible world where messaging or scripting is constant, we are advised simply to stop. Recently, it has become quite trendy to try and stop our distraction. Many books have been written about existing in the now and scheduling, planning, or achieving a goal of regular meditation practice. What ends up happening, however, is that amidst the stress of everything else that's going on around us, we become even more distracted and unfocused. We may end up feeling guilty that we can't keep up with our meditation practice or steady our minds when we do. We may end up blaming ourselves or others for our failures. And then, we may end up as victims of our own failed efforts to meditate on demand, and do it perfectly every time. Perhaps we then use these words: "I know I *should* start meditating, but I just don't have time right now" or "I'm just too busy to stop my life and do this."

We know that existing in a state of constant imbalance (physical, emotional, and even financial) is unhealthy, and we truly desire to become balanced in our lives. But with all of our rules and agendas and the analytical way we approach things, we end up externalizing

OVERVIEW OF THE 7 PRINCIPLES OF HEALTH | 31

the law of balance and turn it into a requirement. And then we try to measure up to some unattainable goal of perfection by noting our every effort: when we think we've succeeded and when we think we have failed. Our belief in this *requirement* to become balanced has us trying to measure up to it and keeping track of how well we're doing in excruciating detail, so much so that it often becomes just another thing we feel we need to do. What's worse, when we don't meet this balance requirement that we've set up for ourselves, we feel guilty. Bewilderingly, Western society has managed to make relaxation, meditation, and becoming centered — things that should make us feel better — a source of inordinate guilt!

Of course, our minds love this instability. Our egos jump from thought to thought, like frolicking monkeys, ceaselessly providing us with even more scripted messaging, phrases like: "I know I should meditate and stop all these thoughts that keep spinning inside my head, but I just can't. I wonder what time I'm supposed to pick up the kids. Oh my, the rent is due, and Josh said he's not going to get his part of our client project finished on time! Why does he do this to me? Our last presentation was a disaster, and Janice chewed me out over it. Oh crap, look what time it is! I just wish I could stop and meditate for a minute, but that's not going to happen any time soon..."

And so it goes.

Principle 1, *Be Present,* helps us realize that our old thought programs take us out of the experience of being inside our bodies, minds, and world, causing us to live inside our heads instead. We find ourselves moving out of the present moment to relive the past or worry about the future. We relinquish our connection to the present and what's actually happening right here and right now. We forget our desire to put quality food in our bodies for nourishment, as we race to work, shoveling fast food into our mouths. We fail to notice the sunshine and cool breeze as we yack on the phone during our morning exercise walk. To truly begin to find health, we must learn how to *Be Present* in this moment — right here and right now. We must learn how to shut down the white noise out there, and quiet ourselves to listen.

32 | THE 7 PRINCIPLES OF HEALTH

PRINCIPLE 2: Become Aware

The second principle is *Become Aware*. Become aware of what?

First, it will be nice to know and experience where we are physically in this world, who we're with, what the day is like, the sounds we're hearing, the flavors we're tasting, and the sensations we're feeling. As odd as it may sound, we often forget to notice the very things that are happening in the present moment. But in terms of *The 7 Principles of Health*, we're also going to need to *Become Aware* of something much more important: our healthcare system and the way it operates to keep us sick.

One key reason we don't know how to become healthy is the programming or scripting we find within our medical system. Essentially, much of this cloak-and-dagger messaging comes from external stakeholders who have much to gain by keeping us in the dark about how the medical machine operates. This includes keeping doctors uninformed about what they're really doing, in terms of trying to help their patients. It is in each of these stakeholders' financial, political, and social best interest to keep us out of the know, blind to seeing a different paradigm.

In spite of these stakeholders' best efforts, however, many people are beginning to realize that something is amiss in healthcare. They're coming to understand that Americans pay a tremendous amount of money for their healthcare system, but rank among the worst in terms of quality of health indicators when compared to other countries that pay much less. Americans are beginning to see that one of the contributing factors to our growing poverty levels is the cost of healthcare. Nevertheless, they still don't understand exactly why we've ended up here.

The next step on our journey to health is to *Become Aware* of another paradigm in healthcare, one that's rooted in fear. We must *Become Aware* of how this messaging is constructed and how it serves to keep us distracted, disempowered, and as victims within the context of our medical system. If we are unaware of this view or fail to understand this seemingly paradoxical statement, we will never be able to find real health. A messaging of fear that promotes victimization will lead only to attempts to counteract the fear and victimization, which will, in turn, lead to more disease.

In the stillness and quiet of being present, we can begin to listen to another voice that teaches us to be aware of what's actually happening around us. And from that new viewpoint, we can begin to make different choices for ourselves.

PRINCIPLE 3: Be Health

Principle 3 is *Be Health*. It does not tell us to *become healthy* or try desperately to *get well soon*. These are future events which may or may not occur and which whisk us away from the present moment: they have not happened yet. While we would like them to happen, once we get pulled into the medical system in an effort to bring about our desired results, we are more likely to fail to find true health. The thought environment not only inside ourselves but inside the system that has taught us to think this way will keep us sick.

When viewing the concept of wellness from a new paradigm, we learn that in order to *become* health, we must start by realizing that we *are* health right now. There is no one, not a single person who is living, who is not health. You may disagree with this statement. You may think that your dad, who's just been diagnosed with terminal pancreatic cancer and has been given only a few months to live, is not in health. But he is in health. Just like Allison, and as you will see with Pastor John, your dad is in health, right here and right now. The question he faces is how he will live before he dies.

It is the act of living every day that will determine our health, not the labels of pancreatic cancer or breast cancer we may receive from our doctors or medical system. It is when we decide how we're going to live before we die, regardless of scripting, messaging, thought forms, or doctors' labels, that we can become medical miracles.

PRINCIPLE 4: Reawaken Curiosity

By nature, we are curious. We love to learn things. Principle 4, *Reawaken Curiosity*, reminds us that we have forgotten how to be curious about our health and helps us reignite that curiosity. There is no end to our learning in every aspect of our lives, including our health.

34 | THE 7 PRINCIPLES OF HEALTH

On our journey to health, we must reawaken our natural sense of inquisitiveness, as it is the very spice of life — and also our path to a healthful one. When we become curious about our bodies and how they work — nothing too fancy, just some interesting, pertinent information — we can use these new facts to teach ourselves. One way we can do this is by seeking out health providers who are passionate about teaching us health practice, and who will show us how to focus on optimal health, rather than disease. They will teach us and help us refocus our attention from the disease preached by most conventionally trained doctors and the medical system, giving us new options for living in health.

By aligning ourselves with Principle 4, we will find that stimulating our perhaps long-dormant curiosity leads us to awakening our own innate ability to heal. We each already posses this skill, no matter how deeply buried it may be under the old scripting; we know this is true because we were all once curious children.

PRINCIPLE 5: Channel Creativity

Health providers who are passionate about healing are not necessarily doctors. They are not the folks who will screen you for cancer or high blood pressure. In Principle 5, *Channel Creativity*, we begin to understand that we are innately creative individuals. When it comes to healthcare, we have allowed our creative abilities to be stifled, which has led to increasing epidemics of disease. But how are the two related? What does lack of creativity have to do with higher rates of disease?

When a disease-focused medical system provides networks of disease-focused health practitioners with an economic incentive to practice disease-focused medicine, what is the only possible result for your personal state of health? Prevention, as you now are aware, is preached at all levels but is rarely practiced because there's no money in it. How can we expect prevention to be practiced when the only practitioners who actually advocate for health are not allowed into your health provider network?

Channeling creativity refers to finding the strength, after mastering the habits underlying Principles 1 through 4, to begin to cre-

OVERVIEW OF THE 7 PRINCIPLES OF HEALTH | 35

ate your own personal health network. The resolve to do so comes from understanding that a different paradigm is possible from which to begin your journey to health. When we understand health, we re-program our thoughts and belief patterns toward health instead of disease, and we begin to manifest health in our lives.

The first manifestation of health shows up in our relationships, the individuals with whom we choose to surround ourselves. We no longer simply go with the disease-focused flow. We no long simply be-lieve what we are told to believe. We no longer do what we are told to do. We begin making healthy choices for ourselves and seek out those experts who view health — not disease — as the starting point. We push away those who start from a disease-focused paradigm into the periphery of our health-focused network. At this stage, we shift even further toward a well-centered, knowledgeable standpoint, aligning ourselves with our very own personal health network, those friends and experts who will stand with us in health.

PRINCIPLE 6: Grow and Renew

One of the natural laws is the law of growth and renewal. We live on a constantly changing planet and exist within a dynamic universe. As hu-mans, we are also constantly changing, from the moment we're born till the moment we die. And yet we struggle to find health within a static system that is based on mechanical theories of fix and cure, test and analyze, diagnose and treat. This is incongruous to our very nature and makes no sense at all. When we get a checkup and come home labeled as "healthy" after our doctor has screened for disease, we're not healthy at all. We are simply free of detectable illness. And that mo-ment after the test results came back has already passed. Poof! — and our moment of health is over. This type of messaging, with which we are all so very familiar, is no way to find health. Health is integrated and dynamic, just the way we were built. In order to find health, we must align ourselves with a different paradigm, one that is also integrated and dynamic.

As we begin to re-program our thoughts toward understanding growth and renewal, surrounding ourselves with providers who prac-tice health this way and who can teach us how to care for ourselves

36 | THE 7 PRINCIPLES OF HEALTH

through dynamic treatments, we will find the balance we seek. This balance, consistent with who we are as humans, will arise from the changing, energetic nature of our very being.

PRINCIPLE 7: Heal, Change, and Thrive

Principle 7 emphasizes that by methodically following the steps and adopting the habits contained in Principles 1 through 6, we will *Heal, Change, and Thrive*. Our goal as humans should be more than mere survival. We want to live great lives. We want to experience such happiness that we glow every day. We want to love the people who surround us and cherish every moment of every day. We want to thrive.

Take a moment to experience a garden. Appreciate the vibrant colors and inhale the fragrant smells. Listen to the incredible sounds of life that buzz around the branches or the wings that beat the air. Nothing in nature simply survives. Nature thrives. It's amazing and it amazes. And, it lives. As an intimate part of it, so must we.

The 5 Disciplines of Health Practice

The 7 Principles of Health are natural, overarching laws we must follow in order to find optimal health. Underlying *The 7 Principles of Health* are five practices, or disciplines. The word discipline means training. We will use these five disciplines to train ourselves for long-lasting health, not unlike training for a marathon. The following is a list of *The 5 Disciplines of Health Practice* without which cannot attain *The 7 Principles of Health*.

1. Releasing Fear

2. Stopping Judgment

3. Letting Go

4. Accepting

5. Practicing Now, Daily, and In Moderation

We can represent *The 5 Disciplines of Health Practice* with the diagram on the next page.

OVERVIEW OF THE 7 PRINCIPLES OF HEALTH | 37

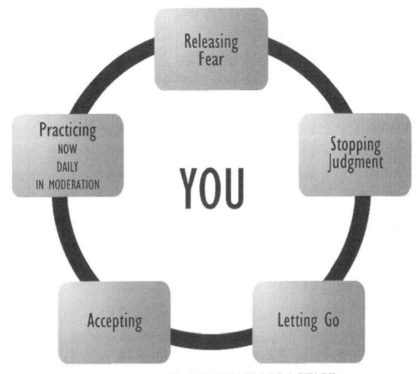

5 DISCIPLINES OF HEALTH PRACTICE

It's fun to imagine that *The 5 Disciplines of Health Practice* are embedded into the shape of a person with his or her arms outstretched. This is the basis for Leonardo Da Vinci's famous Vitruvian Man. At the center of the shape — the figure's heart — is you.

As in the above diagram, *The 5 Disciplines of Health Practice* surround us. They show how we must proceed in order to find health. Let's briefly review each one of these five disciplines.

DISCIPLINE 1: Releasing Fear

At the top of the diagram, in our head, so to speak, is the idea of ***Releasing Fear***. As we are beginning to understand, our present healthcare system was founded on fear. It is not really healthcare that we have, but rather ***health-fear*** that we practice as patients, doctors, and systems. But what are we so afraid of? I believe, quite simply, that we are afraid of the one thing we cannot change or avoid, no matter how hard

38 | THE 7 PRINCIPLES OF HEALTH

we try or how much money we spend. I believe that we are afraid of our own death.

As we discussed in Chapter 1, the International Classification of Diseases (ICD coding system) classifies the causes of death and disease, and we've used this system for more than 200 years. Yet to this day, there is no amount we can pay to have anyone help us avoid our own mortality.

The first discipline we must learn is how to live while facing our fears. We cannot stop ourselves from dying, and trying to ignore or avoid this fact will cause us to sicken and die long before our actual deaths. When we master the concept of *Releasing Fear* with respect to our health, we become able to face our disease challenges with a new attitude that directs us to health, one where we take responsibility for our actions. We begin to understand that what we do or don't do in our health practice directly impacts the outcomes for our minds, bodies, and spirits. When we start to practice releasing our fear as training for our health, we learn to embody it in every aspect of our lives.

DISCIPLINE 2: Stopping Judgment

The right side of the diagram, or left hand of the Vitruvian Man, represents the concept of *Stopping Judgment*. Judgment and opinion infuse almost every aspect of our lives. We judge ourselves. We judge each other. We have opinions about everything and everyone in our world. Our personal judgments can cause a great deal of disagreement and conflict. My opinions or judgments as a doctor, and yours as a patient, can also keep you sick.

For example, if I, as a conventional doctor, have a strong, unfounded opinion about vitamins, supplements, and/or herbal treatments and use derogatory language about them or recommend that you not use those products to promote your own health, I effectively close off options for your potential health and healing. Because I am in a position of relative authority, you may seek my opinion and regard it as that of an expert, which means that my *opinion* could significantly affect your health or lack thereof. You then may find it difficult to disagree with me and make other — perhaps better — choices for yourself. You also might hesitate to pursue alternative treatments which could

OVERVIEW OF THE 7 PRINCIPLES OF HEALTH | 39

have otherwise helped you. The result is that my judgment and I have effectively served to keep you sick, rather than helped you get well.

It's also essential to be aware of your own judgments. Often we are blind to our own polarized opinions and unable to appreciate another's viewpoint. This entire book is about paradoxes and alternate paradigms in healthcare. It is important that you learn to stop judging, proceed with an open mind, and deliberately seek to see things differently. In this way, you will be able to view a bigger picture and you can then choose to take a different direction. Without such an open perspective, your health options are limited, at best.

DISCIPLINE 3: Letting Go

The lower right of the diagram, or the Vitruvian Man's left foot, represents the idea that we need to let go of things in order to heal. Releasing, or *Letting Go*, is a phrase in common use these days. It seems we have so much in our lives to release. But what exactly do we need to let go of when it comes to our health?

We often drag our past with us, well into our golden years. We've been conditioned to live in the past and use it to make excuses. For example, if we are obese as an adult, one of our excuses may be that our parents made us finish all the food on our plates at every meal. But we're here now, in the present; the past and those plates around the family dinner table are long gone. Yet we've carried around that messaging for all these years, allowing it to be our excuse for not changing. If we want to find health, we must have the discipline to let go of the past.

Letting Go, or releasing things, is just as important when we think about the future. In this day and age, it's very normal to worry about future events, especially how we're going to pay for healthcare in America. We worry about getting cancer or some other catastrophic illness and dying, or going bankrupt due to insurmountable medical bills. So we follow the same scripting we've always followed. We pay exorbitant amounts of money for health insurance to protect us from some future event that we are worried about today, an event that has not yet happened.

What if we were to save that money and use it toward health practice today, instead of pouring it into a health insurance sinkhole

40 | THE 7 PRINCIPLES OF HEALTH

for some unknown tomorrow? That nonexistent future event might never happen! But if we continue to spend excessive amounts of money to "insure" against future events which have not yet happened simply because we are afraid they might happen, we are likely to manifest those catastrophic events into our reality because we have been so busy worrying that we failed to take care of our health today!

> "Today is the tomorrow you've been waiting for."
>
> — Anonymous

In order to find true health, we must let go of the past *and* the future. We must not only learn to *Be Present* and *Become Aware*, but release our fears and act in accordance with healing, changing, and thriving. We must exist in this moment called "now" and *Be Health*; with that, we will *Reawaken Curiosity*, *Channel Creativity*, learn how to *Grow and Renew*, and open our innate ability to heal.

DISCIPLINE 4: Accepting

The lower left side of our diagram, or the Vitruvian Man's right foot, represents the discipline of *Accepting*. We must learn how to accept many things in the context of health. The thing with which we seem to have the most trouble is our own mortality. But death, ironically, is the only thing we all must someday face. Learning to accept this fact can lead us back to the present moment. When we are able to acknowledge that we will all die one day, we are then able to ask a much more important question: "How do we want to live in the present?"

I have met many people who were told that chemotherapy, radiation, or surgery would prolong their lives for a few months. They were given no other options by their doctors. During those last few months, they followed their doctors' orders and lived a quality of life unfit for dogs. Then they died.

Accepting our mortality allows us to make a choice about how we want to live within the context of any challenge we face, including something as devastating as terminal cancer. It allows us to stand up for our choices with confidence and shows us that the word *heal* is different than the word cure, and that really there is no *cure*. There is only health.

DISCIPLINE 5. Practicing Now, Daily, and In Moderation

Finally, on the diagram's left upper side, or the Vitruvian Man's right hand, is our daily practice, or our habits. First, we must practice health right here and right now. We cannot wait for some magical future day to begin. For one thing, no such date exists. Have you ever met someone who said, "I've got to clean my house before the housekeeper comes" or "I've got to get in shape before I start going to the gym?" Aren't those ridiculous statements? There is no magical future date when we will be ready to begin being healthy.

Next, we must practice health daily, so that slowly, over time, we begin to live our practice. We become our practice of health. We become healthy. This is not to say that we won't make mistakes or we'll be perfect every time. However, when we develop good habits over an extended period of time and they become second nature, we will slowly, surely, and carefully find health that lasts a lifetime.

Finally, we practice health in moderation and find balance in all aspects of our lives. This means we do a little of everything as it relates to our health: nourishment, exercise, work, leisure, and silence. We don't need to freak out or live in fear, dashing out to run a marathon after having spent the last 20 years on the couch just because our doctor said we have to diet and exercise or we'll die. Let's slow down. Relax a moment. Yes, we will die. That's inevitable. But it doesn't have to be tomorrow. And we don't need to set ourselves up to fail. Begin now to practice health — slowly, deliberately, daily, and in moderation, and soon we will understand how to live well before we die.

Training for health using *The 5 Disciplines of Health Practice* allows us to shift away from disease-focused thinking in every moment to a perspective that begins with health. Every day now becomes an opportunity instead of a difficulty. The diagram on the following page illustrates how a foundation of fear can lead to disease, or a state of extreme *dis*-ease, through our judgments, inability to let go, and refusal to accept things as they are.

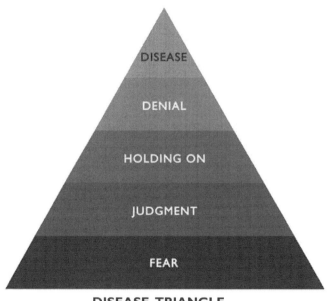

DISEASE TRIANGLE

But, if we begin with a foundation that releases our fear, stops judgment, releases our past and future worries, and accepts things as they are, we can find optimal health or ease in our lives.

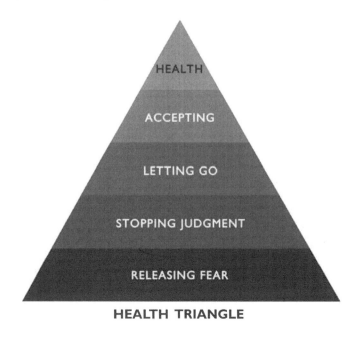

HEALTH TRIANGLE

OVERVIEW OF THE 7 PRINCIPLES OF HEALTH | 43

Our ability to find health is always a direct reflection of the way we view disease. If we view disease as an opportunity, we can reflect that through our state of health, despite the labels conventional medicine and/or our healthcare system might place on us. Disease can become our source of empowerment. The answer lies in the particular paradigm through which we choose to view it. The upcoming story of Pastor John is a perfect example of someone who looked into the mirror of disease and was able to find lasting health.

●

Pastor John sits in the nutrition class where I am a guest speaker. He's 65 years old, with a round belly, rosy cheeks, and a smile that spreads from ear to ear. His eyes are warm and blue as he takes my hand. The comparison to Santa Claus is not misplaced.

"I was given two weeks to live," he tells me. "That was more than five years ago."

Pastor John tells me he was diagnosed with kidney cancer, which had spread to his lungs. He was told he had 28 different cancerous nodules in both lungs, and that chemotherapy and radiation would be useless. His doctors told him to go home and die.

"He was hard, the doctor," Pastor John tells me, his blue eyes clouding over. I ask him what his doctor did after he announced that there was no hope. "He told me my prognosis and then walked to the door, suggesting I go and pick out my coffin."

Pastor John pulls out a set of before-and-after pictures of himself that he carries around with him. He shows me both photos. The one on the left is an image of a pasty, yellow, emaciated man with an oxygen cannula strapped to his face. He looks like a living corpse. The picture on the right shows him as he is today, with his arms wrapped around his beautiful wife of 40 years.

"I did go and pick out my coffin," he says. "They rolled me into the store like this," he taps the picture on the left, "and I remember choosing one."

"What happened?" I ask, incredulous.

"I don't know," he says. "But I received a message that it wasn't time for me to go yet. I was told that I was supposed to stay here and learn how to live."

44 | THE 7 PRINCIPLES OF HEALTH

Today, Pastor John has a website where he's pulled together a community of people. He takes care of himself by eating well, though he pats his belly with a smile, saying, "I know, I still have a few pounds to lose." Most importantly, he gives himself back to the world. He lives for life. He lives for health. He knows what it's like to taste the fear of death and understands what it means to be forced to accept the present as it is and find a new way to live. Once he found the answer, he received a second chance.

Pastor John's wife makes sure that all aspects of his health are managed meticulously. She's his biggest, most vocal fan. She's had to be, in the face of her husband's experience. "I was 20 when I married her," he says. "And she was 19. We've been together ever since."

Was Allison sick? Was Pastor John sick? They each had to ask themselves that question, despite their doctor's prognosis and their disease labels. And both chose to see something very different than what they were *told* to believe.

It's not reacting to the problem but the way we see the problem that's the real answer to finding health.

The 5 Components of Total Health

As you are beginning to see, you must balance many different aspects of life in order to find health. So what are the primary components of health?

Modern medicine has told us that health is the sum of our physical bodies, cognitive or mental capacity, and emotional state. These aspects are represented by the different specialties doctors choose to pursue during the course of their careers. For example, a doctor can become a cardiologist, dermatologist or gastroenterologist, treating the physical diseases that affect those systems. He or she can become a neurologist, treating cognitive or mental disease; or a psychiatrist or psychologist, treating emotional disease. But reducing a complex human being into the study of physical, mental, and emotional states of disease is incomplete.

What about the environment and how it affects our health? What about our spiritual outlook — or lack thereof — or our alignment with the natural gifts and talents that give us a feeling of fulfillment in our lives? Do you think these could be considered as components of total health? Finally, what about our financial stressors and the events in our lives which cause us to worry? Is our financial state of health also a component to our overall state of health?

The 5 Components of Total Health are not only physical, mental or cognitive, and emotional states of health, but also encompass our financial and spiritual aspects. Why? How can our finances determine our health?

As you will come to understand by reading this book, we have deeply eroded our personal finances under the guise of "finding health." Just about everyone in America is out of balance in at least this one aspect. And this imbalance has deeply affected our emotional health, manifesting in ever-increasing rates of anxiety, stress, and fear. This emotional and mental upset has led to a marked increase in physical diseases that are in epidemic proportions according to current health statistics reports.

The culmination of this imbalance and its resulting stressors has caused us to lose faith: in trusting our political systems; in accepting the widening gap between the very rich and the poor; in hope for our environment, which is being sacrificed at every turn; in eking out a place in our struggling economy, with its foundation in greed and profit; and in approaching our personal relationships, reflected by the isolated, selfish ways in which we've come to live. An astonishing number wonder what they are living for. Do we live to run like gerbils on a corporate treadmill, harming others and our world in the name of the all-important bottom line? Or is there a deeper meaning to our existence? The answer to *this* question is the spiritual component of our health and must be in balance with the others if we are to find total health.

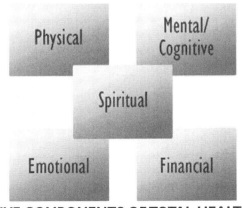

FIVE COMPONENTS OF TOTAL HEALTH

The 7 Requirements for Health Practice

As we have seen, following different disciplines is like implementing a training program. It's great to have discipline, but if we don't also honor certain requirements, we will be only mediocre candidates for our training program and will likely end up failing.

The 7 Requirements for Health Practice can be viewed similarly to the way a job applicant must meet certain criteria for the position. For example, you probably would not want a person to pilot a commercial jetliner with passengers if he or she had never gone to aeronautics school and learned how to fly an airplane. The same applies to your health. There are certain requirements which must be met.

The following is a list of each of *The 7 Requirements for Health Practice*.

1. Desire
2. Commitment
3. Lifelong View
4. Self-Accountability
5. Sequential Steps
6. Small Steps
7. Outside-in, Inside-out

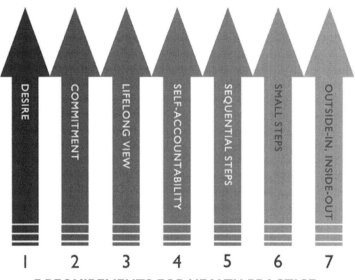

7 REQUIREMENTS FOR HEALTH PRACTICE

OVERVIEW OF THE 7 PRINCIPLES OF HEALTH | 47

REQUIREMENT 1: Desire

Somewhere along the way we adopted the belief that someone else can fix, change, or cure us. This includes holding the healthcare system and doctors responsible for our health. But nothing could be further from the truth. The healthcare system and its doctors cannot make us healthy, even though they promise to do so by using a variety of techniques, including punishment, scolding, nagging, taxes, cost increases, and mandates. We cannot find health if we do not first have Requirement 1, the *Desire* to be health.

My friend works with a healing modality known as quantum energy healing. She has quite a reputation for helping people heal themselves. She told me that one day a man with Parkinson's called her.

"I want you to fix me," he said.

She explained to him that she would do her utmost to help. She would hold his hand through thick and thin and give him the tools to heal, but she would not fix him. He would be the one who would help himself.

"Then I'm not working with you," he said flatly and hung up the phone.

A month later he called her back. "I'm in," he wailed. "I'm getting worse and the doctor's treatments aren't helping."

Who is the only person who can really help you heal? Until you have the *Desire* to help yourself, no one — absolutely no one — can fix you.

REQUIREMENT 2: Commitment

A second requirement for a successful health practice is *Commitment*. If we have the *Desire* but we don't commit to changing for the long term, we won't see any significant results. This doesn't mean we will be perfect in our attempts. It just means that in our *Commitment* to lasting health, we will focus again and again, for the rest of our lives, on health practice. We will commit to recommitting. We will choose whether lasting health is more important to us than eating poorly, avoiding exercise, and stressing out every day. We will make the decision for ourselves because we have chosen life in this present moment. That's the bottom line.

48 | THE 7 PRINCIPLES OF HEALTH

From this deep *Commitment* comes lasting change. Our choices will lead us to health, and we will discover our own ability to heal. This *Commitment* will serve us well in every aspect of life.

REQUIREMENT 3: Lifelong View

Our desire is for health, so we commit to it. We cannot throw away our health and somehow expect to get a second chance. Our health is for life and it is life; it's all we've got. Health is not something we can purchase; nor can we purchase a promise to protect us from death and disease. Similarly, our health is not a liability, as health insurance companies would have us believe. So another requirement for the practice of health is that it requires a *Lifelong View*. It's really that simple.

REQUIREMENT 4: Self-Accountability

We are responsible for ourselves in every avenue of life, including our health. As we have mentioned, no one can fix us in disease — not even doctors. Doctors can help you temporarily cure a very specific condition like bronchitis, but they cannot fix your health.

Self-Accountability is different than *Commitment* or *Desire*. We may desire to lose weight and commit to a practice of eating well, but what happens if we don't find the pounds dropping off? If we don't achieve the weight loss we desire, we may instantly look for someone else to blame — often our spouses or our children. We may make excuses to our doctors and health practitioners as to why we couldn't sustain our health practice, but we know when we're lying to ourselves. We're not fooling our doctors, our spouses, or our kids. All we've done is deceive ourselves into thinking that they believe us because doing so allows us to dodge responsibility for our actions toward our own health practice.

While health providers and our support systems (e.g., family and friends) may go to the ends of the earth to see us succeed in our health goals, we must be accountable to ourselves for that success. We can't find lasting change in health if we do it for others — for our spouses, our children, or our friends. We won't even find it if we do it because our doctors, health insurance companies, lawyers, or the

OVERVIEW OF THE 7 PRINCIPLES OF HEALTH | 49

government demand it. We must do it for ourselves. When we are committed enough in our desire to change, we hold ourselves accountable to our practice because in the end, we are the only ones who matter.

REQUIREMENT 5: Sequential Steps

We must follow *The 7 Principles of Health* in sequence if we are to truly shift our perspective about health. It's not possible to succeed if we skip any of these steps. We can cut corners, perhaps believing that we've quickly mastered each principle, but we'll soon discover an interesting truth. In order to open to our innate source of health and healing, we must take each of *The 7 Principles* in order so that we can discern where we are within our current health paradigm. Just like laying bricks to build a house, we cannot put the last brick in place until a strong foundation has already been built.

REQUIREMENT 6: Small Steps

Health and healing are found by taking small steps, one at a time. When the medical profession dictates orders to us, like "Diet and exercise!" we often don't know where to begin. We erroneously believe we must shrink to a Size 6 within a month of our new practice, so we follow false promises which often make us sicker than ever before. This reminds me of an advertisement I saw recently for bariatric surgery (stomach stapling). The ad promised you'd shrink by one pound a day, *without* any diet or exercise. What's wrong with this promise? Health doesn't work that way! Health is the result of a *Lifelong View* and the pursuit of lasting change, and it can be overwhelming for our entire system to attempt to achieve it all at once.

But if we break down big tasks or projects into small parts, performing them one step at a time without necessarily focusing on our difficult overall goal, we get there anyway without trying so hard. Instead of seeking the quick fix, we must focus on the intent of our practice. The intent of a health practice is to live optimally. And we live optimally in health inside every moment of our life, making conscious choices for our next meal, hydration, exercise, play, or action. We learn *The 7 Principles of Health*, *The 5 Disciplines of Health Practice*, and

The 7 Requirements for Health Practice, seeking to practice each, in turn, every day in order to find our way to optimal health. These small steps then become our health practice, which becomes our daily habits, which subsequently lead us to optimal health without attaching to difficult or esoteric goals. And, paradoxically, this practice helps us safely, steadily, and effectively attain all our goals.

REQUIREMENT 7: Outside-in, Inside-out

Many people believe that in order to affect change, for example in the workplace or at home, we must begin from within. *The 7 Principles of Health*, however, are approached from the outside, and proceed inward.

Why do we need to start like this?

In the context of medicine today, I believe the only way for each of us to find health and

> *"Fears are educated into us, and can, if we wish, be educated out."*
>
> **— Karl Augustus Menninger**

learn how to heal is by proceeding from the outside-in to unlearn the disease-focused messages we have been taught to believe. The problem is that we've been steeped in a single mindset for so long that we have constructed an entire system around these beliefs. We've been so ingrained about how to think and act that we have become unable to see any other perspective. The weight of conventional medical thought keeps us well entrenched inside the boxes we have created for ourselves. Thus we continue to perpetuate those belief systems, spending more and more money every year, without changing our thinking in any way.

In order to uncover our innate ability to heal, we must proceed then, from the *Outside-in*. When we do it this way, we begin to understand how we came to embrace our current perspective, or what I call the "currency" of disease-focused medicine. We must start with the concepts, words, and viewpoints that are so familiar to us, breaking them down little by little, so that an altogether different viewpoint is presented.

As we build our knowledge, skills, and practice, our perspectives will organically shift — we won't have to force it because it will

OVERVIEW OF THE 7 PRINCIPLES OF HEALTH | 51

happen naturally. We will find that we can hold a different view of health and healing. Concurrently, as we proceed to apply Principles 1 through 7, ultimately arriving at the inner circle in the center of the diagram of *The 7 Principles of Health*, we will reach our own core of healing strength. Like Allison and Pastor John, both of whom were challenged with extremely difficult diagnoses and decided to change the way they regarded the medical system and their own health, we will learn to shift our mindset before it's too late.

Our healthcare system, with its medical providers, dogma, training and education, systems, institutions, and viewpoints, was constructed to result in sick, aging, and unhealthy individuals. If you want to find health inside its confines, that is, if you truly want to heal, you will have to find the strength to stand up against much of the system and its components, learn to see things differently, and begin making your own choices.

The View from Outer Space

I'd like to end this overview with a view from outer space, perhaps one of the biggest-picture views we can take using our current technology. World famous astronomer, the late Carl Sagan, showed us just how fragile our planet is.

> Consider again that dot. That's here. That's home. That's us. On it everyone you love, everyone you know, everyone you ever heard of, every human being who ever was, lived out their lives. The aggregate of our joy and suffering, thousands of confident religions, ideologies, and economic doctrines, every hunter and forager, every hero and coward, every creator and destroyer of civilization, every king and peasant, every young couple in love, every mother and father, hopeful child, inventor and explorer, every teacher of morals, every corrupt politician, every 'superstar,' every 'supreme leader,' every saint and sinner in the history of our species lives there — on a mote of dust suspended on a sunbeam.

I hope this book will help you understand just how fragile we are as humans. Over the last century, we've abused our homes — not only

52 | THE 7 PRINCIPLES OF HEALTH

our beautiful planet which sustains our life, but our bodies as well. Yet we live during an age of tremendous change. Modern society and its greed-, profit-, and power-based belief systems are taking their toll on our population. We are being pulled apart, as the gap between the haves and the have-nots widens.

Likewise, these attitudes of greed and profit in our healthcare system form a crumbling foundation that is affecting all of us. We witness this in the increasing number of preventable diseases that have reached epidemic proportions. As conscious individuals, however, we are beginning to understand that our bodies, minds, finances, emotions and spirits are being systematically destroyed.

After learning *The 7 Principles of Health*, you will come to realize that you now have a choice. You will walk away with the power to make your own health decisions. You will have the ability to choose to regain your personal power and begin to stand up against a system that wants to keep you ill for its own purposes and profits. You will be able to do this, no matter where your starting point is — disease or no disease — it doesn't matter. These are merely labels, as you will soon come to understand.

As patients, it will be vitally important to save ourselves by changing our perspectives. We cannot wait for our political or medical systems to do this for us. As doctors, we must shift our own paradigms and confront ourselves, our egos, our judgments, and our myopic training bias that is rooted in disease. We must learn to stop practicing medicine under the old dogma and learn how to collaborate with many other healers and health practitioners. We must learn how to practice health, just like our patients.

I invite you to come along on this journey and open yourself to your own amazing potential to heal, a long-forgotten gift that has lain dormant for so many years.

CHAPTER THREE

Principle 1
Be Present

"In the midst of movement and chaos, keep stillness inside of you."
— **Deepak Chopra, M.D.** *(b. 1946)*
Indian-born American physician and author

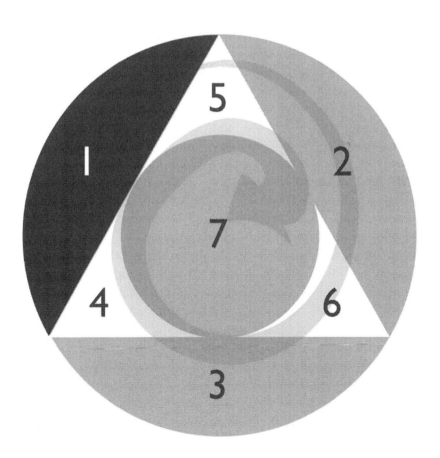

54 | THE 7 PRINCIPLES OF HEALTH

Have you ever noticed the bright yellow boxes hanging on the walls in many public places like airports and gymnasiums? The box has a picture of a lightning bolt on its cover. This box contains a piece of medical equipment called an Automated External Defibrillator, or AED. We use it to jumpstart a person's heart when they collapse from a heart attack. It works by sending an electrical current through erratically beating cells, "stunning" them. The AED allows the heart to take something of a timeout moment and reorganize. During this brief time, the heart stops beating and the person is effectively dead.

It may seem counterintuitive to save a person's life by stopping their heart. However, if we don't stop the chaotic rhythm caused by those crazy electrical impulses, the patient won't survive. The longer the heart attack victim remains in this chaotic rhythm, or "ventricular fibrillation" as doctors call it, the less chance he or she has of survival. In other words, waiting too long before stopping a victim's heart with an AED often results in death.

A fibrillating heart can be compared to sitting on the bleachers during a football game. Many sounds bombard our eardrums at the same time: the shouting crowds, the announcer, loud music, singing buskers, dancing cheerleaders, and the angry guy with the painted face sitting next to you. If you tried to pay full attention to each one of these separate sounds, you'd get whiplash. You wouldn't truly be able to experience each, because you'd be distracted by the next one that was a little louder, and the next after that. You'd get a collection of sound bites, within which you, sitting on the bleachers, would exist.

The AED, by releasing an electrical current to shock all the heart cells at once, would be like a deafening explosion going off in the middle of the football game. It would shut everyone up, at least momentarily. A space would be created during which there was no sound. There would be a brief timeout. The same is true of a hearts that has been defibrillated; the electrical current from the AED basically wipes out all prior chaotic signals and creates a tiny space of time during which nothing happens.

When it comes to healthcare, there's a lot of noise out there in the form of chaotic bits of information or sound bites. Information comes to us through just about every form of communication possible: podcasts, Internet, television, radio, magazines, journals, text mes-

PRINCIPLE 1: BE PRESENT | 55

sages, email, and more. There's virtually no end to the messages about what we need to do to get healthy. Interestingly, each tiny bit of information seems to come with an overall promise of health. For example, you might have heard that eating asparagus can ward off cancer. So you may rush off to the grocery store and buy a bushel of asparagus. You may then cook it up and eat it with each meal every day for the next several until you're eating so much asparagus that you're sure you're turning green.

A few weeks later, you then hear in the news that lemons are sure to stop you from getting cancer. So you stop buying asparagus and pick up a truckload of lemons. You vow to eat lemons six times a day for the rest of your life. But while you've been busy eating asparagus and lemons all those weeks, you may also have been ordering lunch out at work: double-decker cheeseburgers and fries, Kentucky Fried Chicken®, Frappucinos® with whipped cream and chocolate sprinkles, or Arby's® roast beef sandwiches with curly fries. The last sound bite of health information still echoing in your mind was the message that lemons prevent cancer. Since you're *also* eating those every day, just as you've been told, you feel sure you're doing all that's needed to prevent the dreaded illness. It's not long, however, until you can't stand the sight, smell, or taste of lemons. Lemon cake seems much better. You give up your promise to eat lemons and soon forget about preventing cancer.

The truth is that no amount of asparagus or lemons will prevent cancer if, in the grand scheme of things, your foods are laden with saturated fats. We've become so buried in sound bites and details which promise to improve our health or prevent disease that many of us miss the bigger picture.

Perhaps you disagree. Perhaps you believe that health information, as it's currently delivered to us, is very important and that it has helped change our behavior for the better. I agree that it is important and that it has helped many people. But the way our technology, science, and research deliver this information to the average person is, paradoxically, keeping us from finding true health. It keeps us distracted and searching outside ourselves for something that will fix us or help us stay well. It doesn't teach us how to truly help ourselves. We're left to figure that out on our own.

56 | THE 7 PRINCIPLES OF HEALTH

The constant flow of tiny sound bites of health and medical information keeps us inside the box of a medical system that needs us to be sick so that we remain dependent on its components to provide us with healthcare. It polarizes complementary and alternative medicine practitioners against each other and pits patients against their doctors. It keeps us from rising above all the noise and really finding a different way to do things. What we need right now in order to begin a personal journey to health, just like a stricken person's fibrillating heart, is a moment of silence.

Principle 1 helps us to **Be Present**. We need to defibrillate. We need to stop. We need to create space. We need to take time out to learn, once again, how to heal. This is the first step on that journey.

YOUR INVITATION TO PRACTICE HEALTH

I invite you now to focus on being present. Believe it or not, the reason many people give for not stopping for the *single moment* it would take for this most important paradigm shift — a shift that could change their entire lives — is that they just don't have time. Perhaps this has been your reason. It's not very difficult to stop the noise, however. You can do it right now, with very little effort.

Take a moment to read and answer the questions below.

1. Where are you right now? Are you inside a building or outdoors? What colors do you see? Are they bright, dull, textured, or smooth?

2. What do you hear going on around you? Do you hear the sounds of other people? Is it quiet? Do you hear traffic? What about the sound of birds or buzzing insects or the sound of the wind in the leaves?

3. What do you smell? Is someone having a barbeque? Is your house scented with your favorite essential oils? Are you wearing perfume or cologne?

4. What do you feel? Is the sun warm on your face? Are you comfortable? Do you feel safe, cozy, or perhaps another emotion?

PRINCIPLE 1: BE PRESENT | 57

5. What do you taste? Are you sipping a glass of cucumber water or a diet Coke? Are you eating some crackers? Do you feel the hard crunch in your mouth?

●

Like an AED, we must take this moment of silence to find health, but doing so may seem counterintuitive. We may feel we won't be able to fight our diseases if we stop for just a single second. We may be afraid not to do everything our doctors have told us because if we don't, we'll get sick and die. We may be facing terminal diagnoses that are causing immense anxiety and stress in our lives and feel that doing something — anything — is better than doing nothing. We may feel that we need to take care of ourselves *right now*, and that if we don't "do something," we won't heal.

For a brief moment, let's take a step away from our discussion of change in our personal health via *doing* and look at change in a different context. As you read the following examples of remarkable people, consider how each has gone on to change the world in a profound way by first entering a period of silence. Within that space, each was able to create in their minds a different perspective from which they could then operate. From that new paradigm, not only did they change themselves, but they changed their world.

Around 400 B.C., Siddhartha Gautama, the Buddha, taught his followers that silence was the path to enlightenment and freedom. In the West, the teachings of Jesus Christ helped show us that the way to find God is simply by being still. In the silence and stillness of her physical disabilities, Helen Keller, who was born blind and deaf, graduated from Radcliff College and became a prolific author, activist, and humanitarian. In India, Mahatma K. Gandhi was jailed for his views and periodically retreated into long periods of fasting and silence, which became the foundation of his nonviolent movement, and which helped free his country from British rule. Despite being sent to jail for his views on civil rights, Martin Luther King, Jr. was instrumental in desegregating our nation. And finally, Nelson Mandela was held behind bars for many years but still freed his people from the oppression of Apartheid in South Africa.

58 | THE 7 PRINCIPLES OF HEALTH

What do these individuals, who were instrumental in reshaping the world around them, have to do with finding health? I believe that finding our way to healing and health is no different than what each of them did for their country and people. When we stop distracting ourselves with what others tell us — the noise around us — and refocus our full attention toward ourselves, we open a pathway to our own innate ability to heal. We begin to understand the messages that surround us and whether they contain useful information or are simply more chatter. We can set aside the details that serve only to continue to distract us from our underlying purpose of finding optimal health. We stop overeating asparagus and lemons and learn how to balance nourishment, a practice which will last us for the rest of our lives.

The strange thing is, when we begin to see a bigger picture and learn how to heal as individuals first, we begin to care about others and their welfare, too. We begin to care about the future, the world we are leaving behind for our children, and the quality of their future food and water supplies. We find that we cannot help but change our world in profound ways, just like the amazing individuals mentioned above.

In order to find personal health and change, we must first stop distracting ourselves with sound bites of health advice, at least for a moment, and reset. But in order to do this, we need to understand what it takes to change.

●

"Oh, doctor! I'm glad it's you!" The 19-year-old man's eyes are wild with happiness.

"Why?" I ask suspiciously.

"I wanted to thank you! You were the only one who helped me! Don't you remember?"

"Ah ... I see a lot of patients. I'm not sure I remember you, exactly," I reply honestly.

"That's okay. Oh, I'm so glad you're here today. I get to thank you personally."

"What for?"

"I've been clean for a year! I haven't done any drugs. And you were the one who told me how."

PRINCIPLE 1: BE PRESENT | 59

"Um ... what precisely did I tell you?" I ask, trying hard to remember.

He grins from ear to ear, his spiked blond hair sticking out in every direction, like sparks from a firecracker. "You helped me stop doing drugs. You told me to be true to myself. I wanted to thank you. No one has ever told me that before."

"Oh. Did I give you the 'look into the mirror' speech?"

"Yes!" He bursts out laughing. "You did! And you changed my life! You did it, you changed me and I want to say thank you."

"I didn't do anything," I say, smiling at his enthusiasm. "You did it all by yourself. I'm just glad you did."

●

Between the stimulus and the action lies a gap. Inside this gap lies choice. The power to choose and determine our own outcomes is what leads to profound change.

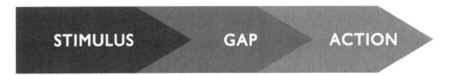

Who is the only person who can change you? Can a doctor force you to get healthy? Can a health insurance company threaten you with escalating costs if you don't stay healthy and then deny coverage when you don't? Can a government mandate you to become healthy or else? In the short term, these punitive measures may work. But the results won't last.

By the year 2016, America's cost of healthcare will be approximately $3.5 trillion and $4.8 trillion by 2021[3]. In 1960, the average per person cost was $147, which then increased to $8,402 by 2010, and $14,103 by 2021. Between January 2000 and January 2012, the median annual household income decreased from $54,790 in 2000 to $50,020 in 2012[4]. Americans today pay almost 45 percent of their earned income toward healthcare costs. All the promises in the world

---

[3]National Health Expenditures Aggregate, Per Capita Amounts, Percent Distribution, and Average Annual Percent Change: Selected Calendar Years, 1960 -2010. Accessed online at http://www.cms.gov.

[4]Green, Gordon and Coder, John. Household income trends: January 2012, Issued March 2012. Sentier Research, LLC. 2012

60 | THE 7 PRINCIPLES OF HEALTH

by external parties can *never* compensate for the underlying fact that we can ever be fixed by any of them. And so the same issues regarding our personal health will arise again and again, because lasting change has not happened from within each of us as individuals. We keep expecting someone else to do it for us. But really, we are the only ones who can help ourselves.

Distraction Eliminates Personal Choice

If we are to choose, we must have the power to do so. But the many distractions surrounding healthcare actually lead to disempowerment, which can be defined as removing authority from the individual and placing it in the hands of someone or something else. When we are highly distracted, focusing our attention on something external, that distraction has power over us. In the earlier examples of asparagus and lemons, we focused our attention on these items as preventive agents for cancer, and that idea had power over us. Our focus on lemons and asparagus diminished our power to view the big picture of health and to choose healthy, balanced meals. We chose Kentucky Fried Chicken® and Arby's® lunches instead, empowered by the belief that asparagus and lemons could still prevent us from getting sick.

Now, imagine all the health advice sound bites out there:

- Take vitamin E.
- Drink six cups of coffee a day.
- Consume two ounces of red wine at night.
- Take this new pill to shrink your fat cells.
- Eat more bok choy, cruciferous vegetables, turmeric, paprika, magnesium, vitamin D3, mulberry extract, ginger, zinc, selenium, green tea, garlic, etc.

The list is endless. Every day we hear some new trick, tip, or tool that guarantees to improve our health. It's no longer possible to follow each separate bit of advice without first grounding ourselves and clearing some space to discover a new paradigm. The problem is that it can be quite difficult to see a new perspective from inside the context of our current paradigm.

PRINCIPLE 1: BE PRESENT | 61

Our medical system does not provide us with tools for significant behavior modification success or guidance from which to form a health perspective. It intentionally limits our power to choose. It provides us, instead, with more and more distracting information, mostly about disease or the threat of disease, death, and dying. The current healthcare system keeps us focused on our struggle to find cure after cure for disease, but it doesn't offer us a way to see beyond disease into our innate ability to heal. Once again, our focus shifts away from health toward disease, which then affects our personal ability to focus on our goal: lasting health. As a result, disease has power over us because we are consumed by thoughts of it. And so again, we wind up back inside The Current Health Paradigm, as referred to in Part I.

This paradigm shift we seek must come back to us, as individuals. Will we choose to focus on multiple distractions like disease and health-messaging sound bites, thereby decreasing our power of personal choice in health? Or will we shift? If we don't learn to stay inside the gap of being present, the only place where we can listen and think clearly about our health choices, we will continue to move on to the next best tip we hear, the next best idea to try, and we will never find the true health for which we were so desperately searching in the first place.

One of my patients recently told me that she's "sick of numbers, graphs, and data. Just tell me like it is, doctor. Tell me the truth."

But what is the truth? We now know more about medicine and health than we've ever known in our history. But we, both as a nation and as global citizens, are getting sicker and sicker in epidemic proportions. We all know the truth; it's contained in health statistics readily available to anyone who cares to read them. But even those statistics added to the white noise of healthcare, serving to do nothing more than keep us highly distracted.

At this point, we really don't need doctors and experts to tell us how to get healthy. We know how — it's just common sense. If we need it, there's plenty of information out there to help us make our own decisions and begin living our own truth on our journey to health. What we need is validation for making these decisions and for reclaiming our power of choice over our own health. We need to become empowered to choose health. To arrive at this concept in spite

62 | THE 7 PRINCIPLES OF HEALTH

of so much distraction, we begin by being present. In order to find our way back to health, to stop fibrillating as chaotically as we have been for as long as we have been, we must first be prepared to metaphorically die for a moment.

●

What causes all this distraction and disempowerment in healthcare?

My friend David lives in Australia. He's 48 years old. He rides his bike, surfs the big waves almost every day, takes Pilates classes to stay toned, and swims. He eats healthy foods and enjoys life. He'd never even seen a doctor until he blew his knee out one day and had to have surgery. A few years later, he wanted to go back to his primary care doctor for a referral to a specialist.

"You're in the demographic of men who never see doctors," said the general practitioner. "You need to go for these tests," the doctor told him, handing him a list of medical exams.

"But I just want a referral to the orthopedic surgeon who operated on my knee. Why do I need all these tests, mate?"

"To determine whether you're healthy. What if you have a problem?"

I asked David how he felt when he went home after his visit with his GP.

"I started to worry that something was wrong with me," he said. "You know, you go home and stew about possibilities, thinking you might have cancer or a big prostate or something like that. And then you worry and worry and it drives you crazy, all this worrying."

●

While it's very important to screen for disease conditions for which early detection has proven benefits (e.g., the Pap test for cervical cancer, colonoscopies for colon cancer, mammography for breast cancer, and blood pressure screening for hypertension), we've gone way overboard in our fervor to rely on testing and screening procedures as the definition of health. The definition of healthy nowadays has become a punch line: someone who hasn't had enough tests. Unfortunately, the message which got downloaded to patients is this: *If the test is negative,*

PRINCIPLE 1: BE PRESENT | 63

you can relax — you're healthy. That is an incorrect assumption, though. The definition of health is not merely the absence of disease. The absence of disease is the absence of disease and nothing more.

The bad news is that doctors have also come to interpret health using this same definition. As in David's example above, his doctor's underlying interpretation, by virtue of his training and paradigm inside a disease-focused system, is that David is not a healthy person unless he has a bunch of negative tests. He tells David that there might be something wrong with him, so David then goes home worried, becoming afraid of the possibility of disease. He begins to dwell on the past and worry over future nonevent situations or illusions. Fear has been introduced into his personal definition of health and now becomes the heart of his ensuing distraction and disempowerment.

Of course, all of this is unintentional. Doctors like me don't intend to introduce fear when we perform the jobs for which we've been educated. For the most part, we are well-meaning individuals who initially went into medicine to help people and try to help them become healthier. But what we weren't able to see is the paradox of a healthcare system that trains us to carry out our jobs by focusing on disease. We didn't question what we were inadvertently teaching our patients through subtly scripted messages shrouded in disease mentality. We just thought we were doing a damn good job.

●

"Your tests are abnormal again. Have you been taking your medication like I told you?" Melissa's doctor asks her.

"I've been trying, Doctor," Melissa says. "But I'm so tired all the time. Why do I feel like this?"

"It's because you're not taking your medication. If you would do what I told you to do and take your meds, you'd feel better. Remember, you are *sick*."

●

Is Melissa really sick? Does she need to be labeled as a sick person, someone who is abnormal, and someone with problems? Or can she simply be Melissa, who has a few health challenges she needs to address?

64 | THE 7 PRINCIPLES OF HEALTH

Nearly three-quarters (73 percent) of our population is overweight or obese. Three hundred sixty million persons worldwide, approximately the entire population of the United States, have type 2 diabetes. Are these people all abnormal? What is normal anymore, when the vast majority of our population is abnormal and sick by our current definitions?

Michael is David's friend. His parents died at a young age: his father contracted tetanus after a wound became infected, and his mother died suddenly in a car accident. An orphan for most of his life, Michael began to fear his own death, so he learned to rely on doctors to tell him that he's healthy.

"My back is sore," he says to David.

"Why don't you see the physiotherapist to help strengthen it?" David replies.

"No. I think I'll see the doctor, just to make sure nothing's wrong."

"What about a chiropractor? I know someone who might be able to help your back. He's really good, this guy."

"No," says Michael. "I'd better book an appointment with my GP."

David explains that Michael has called him with the same story again and again for years. It's almost as if David's friend is in a state of paralysis that's caused by fear of death and disability, and he needs the authority of a doctor to tell him he'll live. To him, a doctor is like a priest, someone who can take away his anxiety and fear of death. But relief is only temporary. As soon as another symptom crops up, he's back in the doctor's office, sick with worry again.

Fear is paralyzing. It strips away our choice, as patients and as doctors. It eliminates our power to choose health, because the default condition always is disease.

●

"Your margins on the breast cancer aren't clear," the surgeon tells Patricia, a patient of mine.

"What does that mean?" she asks.

"Well, we'll have to book you for another surgery. I'd like to make sure we clear out what's left behind and strip down a few more lymph nodes."

PRINCIPLE 1: BE PRESENT | 65

"Are there any other options?"

"You could choose not to have the surgery," he says with a sarcastic tone. "But I wouldn't advise it."

"I don't want to have the surgery," she says firmly.

"What do you mean you don't want to have the surgery? That's a death sentence, what you're saying right now," the doctor says, clearly annoyed.

"I want to find another way, a natural treatment."

"That's ridiculous!" He's unable to contain his outburst. "There's no natural way to treat breast cancer! Here, book your surgery with my secretary." Patricia says the doctor took her by the arm and walked her to the front desk, where his secretary was ready to book her an appointment. She refused and walked out of the surgeon's office.

Patricia then decided to take her health into her own hands. She began talking with friends about eating nourishing foods, drinking quality water, and creating a healthy intracellular environment (the environment inside which a cell exists in our bodies) which would reduce toxicity and lead to healthy cells, not cancerous ones. Her journey was difficult, she tells me. She had no support from her conventional doctors. She says they seemed afraid to recommend anything other than traditional cancer regimens. But she persisted on her own and explains that she's never felt better, especially after deciding for herself.

Fear

Fear lies not only at the heart of distraction and disempowerment in our patients, but also in our own actions as health providers. When we are all disempowered under The Current Health Paradigm, one that's built on disease and fear, we doctors provide recommendations and treatments, seemingly intended to help our patients find health. However, the goal of our treatments is really to help them rid themselves only of those one or two particular diseases. There is no overall plan for optimal health; there is only a monstrous problem list, which for some people can extend to 10 or 15 different medical diagnoses. Following those diagnoses, plans are formulated to attack each problem independently, rather than creating an overall plan to support total optimal health. Ironically, a strategic plan to first nourish and exercise the whole individual will, in many cases, control, reverse, or eliminate all of the diagnosed diseases!

But we're afraid of consequences, too. We're afraid to contradict a multitrillion dollar system, with its regulations and bureaucracy that instill fear of repercussions, mostly economic and legal. We're afraid to get sued. We're afraid to get banned as Medicare providers or prevented from participating in health insurance networks, although we may have done nothing wrong except try and be good doctors. So we practice with this ever-present fear at the back of our minds. As a result of our own personal fears, and operating within this illogical system, we inadvertently keep our patients sick — all under the guise of delivering healthcare.

●

My brother is an emergency room doctor in New Zealand, and he's had the opportunity to see and help patients from many different cultural backgrounds, including those from the Maori tribes. He told me of an interesting discussion he's had with both patients and doctors.

"When sick patients come into the emergency room, I offer them treatment, but unless they're very ill, I encourage them to treat themselves at home. I send most of my cases home. Yet it's amazing how many people actually want to be admitted to the hospital. It's almost as if they believe the hospital is a magical place, and by admission to it, they will be cured. So I've become known amongst the other doctors as 'the guy who doesn't like to admit.'

"I find it funny that most doctors don't stop to think for a minute," he continues. "More than 20 percent of infections in our hospital are nosocomial (found only inside hospitals and not out in the community). This means that a patient admitted to the hospital for any reason stands a greater chance of contracting a resistant strain of a bug that's going to be very difficult to treat. And we're running out of drugs to use against these bugs. But my colleagues seem to think that we should be admitting ambulatory patients. So it begs the question: Are we admitting patients for their sake, or ours?"

How did we become so afraid to heal ourselves without relying on our so-called magical institutions? Modern medicine has transferred

PRINCIPLE 1: BE PRESENT | 67

the idea and expectation of healing to the hospital and, ironically, with this shift we have created *more* disease. We are now facing super-bugs for which we are running out of treatment options. Though we keep trying to cure and fix health problems, as the years go by, the illnesses and conditions become more and more difficult to treat. Yet we persist in promoting hospital admission by virtue of our disease-focused paradigm.

●

"What happened, Dr. Duncan?" My colleague is lying in a hospital bed recovering from a bowel infection. He has a nasogastric tube sticking out of his nose, and he's hooked up to intravenous bags with bright fluorescent stickers all over them, antibiotics to treat the infection.

"I developed pneumonia and then an ileus (intestinal infection) after the operation. They started with ceftriaxone for the pneumonia, but had to go to (intravenous antibiotic drugs) levofloxacin (brand name, Levaquin®) and vancomycin when they found it was resistant."

"But it was supposed to be an outpatient procedure. You just went in for your knee!" I exclaim.

"Post-operative complications. And a nosocomial infection," he says.

"Did you really need to have the knee replaced?" I ask. "I gave you the article on osteoarthritis and acupuncture for knee joints from the NCCAM (National Center for Complementary and Alternative Medicine). Did you check it out?"

Dr. Duncan is the same doctor who refers to our acupuncturist as a "voodoo" practitioner.

We seem always to drive straight toward the disease-fix-cure paradigm, and Dr. Duncan is among the first to recommend such treatment. But what happens when modern medicine runs out of answers for sick individuals?

●

"Hi Don. How can I help you?" I open the door to Exam Room #3. A dejected, worn-out man in his forties sits in the chair; his stomach is bigger than a pregnant woman in her third trimester who's carrying twins. Don is yellow, sallow, and very mellow.

"I don't know, Doc," he says in a thin voice. "I don't have money. I can't get insurance."

"What's your diagnosis?" I ask.

"I've got hepatitis C. I'm terminal, they tell me." He laughs without humor. "It's probably from some tattoo when I was young. I never did drugs and I've been married for 20 years. I just got dealt a bad card, I guess. But I'm in pain, Doc. I try not to use the drugs, but I can't..." He winces at the memory of pain.

"Which drug works for you?" I ask.

"Percocet®." He closes his eyes, as if anticipating my answer. "But the doctors think I'm a drug addict. It's not fair, you know. They won't see me. I'm in real pain — I don't want to be a drug addict — but I'm waiting for a liver transplant."

"How are you going to pay for it?"

He shakes his head. "I don't know. I don't ... I can't get insurance. I'm losing my job. They won't insure me, and I don't qualify for the state plan. My wife earns too much. I came in here with my last bit of cash just to get some pain relief. What do you think I should do?"

I don't reply. I can't. All I want to say is, "I don't know anymore, Don. I don't have any answers for you. I'm so sorry. Maybe you should go home to die."

●

The healthcare tragedy that results from medicine's blind dictates is illustrated through the stories of Don, Patricia, Allison, and Pastor John. What happens when medicine shows us just one side of the coin, and we take its advice in blind faith, only to discover too late that there might have been a different choice?

Fear has led us to forget what matters most: our personal lives and our health; our patients' lives and their health; and our power to change a system that's causing us to freefall, unchecked, into becom-

PRINCIPLE 1: BE PRESENT | 69

ing victims of the very thing we want most, freedom from disease. The way we see the problem is, indeed, our problem. I encourage you now to begin the process of changing your mind's inner attitudes. You can start by *Being Present* in health.

YOUR INVITATION TO PRACTICE HEALTH

Many people make the excuse that they just don't have time to meditate. They tell me, "I know I should, but..." They tell me they're going to start as soon as they get some free time. Many others say they can't meditate, they don't know how, or that it's too hard. But meditation or even just relaxation is really very easy, and it can be done right here, right now. There are only two things you must do to practice Principle 1, *Be Present*, and begin your journey to health:

1. Start

2. Start now

Shall we begin? First, read the following section down to where it says START NOW! and set your watch or timer for one minute.

- After reading the section, close this book or put down your electronic reader.
- Start the timer and close your eyes.
- Take a deep breath in for a count of three.
- Focus on your breath.
- Hold your breath for one count.
- Breathe out for a count of three.
- Focus on your breath.
- Repeat this breathing pattern 5 times.
- If a thought enters your mind, notice it, saying "I am thinking a thought," and push the thought out of your mind.
- Return to your breathing.
- START NOW!

70 | THE 7 PRINCIPLES OF HEALTH

How do you feel? Are you worried about anything? If so, notice whether your worry is about a past event or about a future situation that has not occurred. Does thinking about the past or the future help you focus on the present?

If you didn't stop to do the exercise and simply continued reading past it, ask yourself why you did not stop for one minute to *Be Present*. Did you have a good reason? Or was your reason really just an excuse?

It's okay to have a reason for not trying this first exercise. Be honest at this point — no one is judging you. But understand that if you have time to read this book, you have time to stop and *Be Present*. We will talk a bit later about blame, judgment, and the excuses that ultimately prevent us from empowering ourselves. Just understand that if you truly want to find health in the middle of such a highly distractible society, with its constant noise, it will be necessary to stop — right here, right now. The choice to do so will be yours. Remember, no one else stands in your path to health and no one else can make the changes for you. It's all up to you.

> *"Human beings, by changing the inner attitudes of their minds, can change the outer aspects of their lives."*
>
> — **William James**

If you have a moment, check out more on how to develop a regular practice of becoming silent, and stopping the noise of society's programmed messages by visiting our website at health-conscious.org. You will find a simple record that you can keep by your computer or nightstand to remind you to stop and breathe, even if it's for one minute a day. Every day, you can dedicate this period to personal silence. That's all! At the end of the minute, you can note your progress for the day without getting too fancy - just a simple check-mark in the box. The exercise is not designed to be difficult and may even seem ridiculously simple. It's not, though. The goal is to see if you can become more conscious of practicing regularly for 30 days and then turn this one minute into a priority. Remember, one simple minute a day of silence can lead to optimal health for the rest of your life — I guarantee it!

All you have to do is start now.

CHAPTER FOUR

Principle 2
Become Aware

"We doctors have taken this medicine stuff into the people until they believe it."

— **Ernst Schweninger, M.D.** *(1850-1924)*
Dermatologist and personal physician to German Chancellor Otto von Bismarck

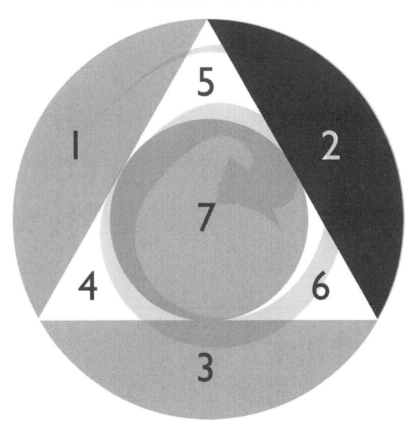

72 | THE 7 PRINCIPLES OF HEALTH

Take a moment to recall the yellow box with the lightning strike hanging on the wall. This is the Automated External Defibrillator (AED) that has just stopped or "defibrillated" our patient's heart. Right now, there's no electrical current and his heart isn't beating. His body is experiencing a placc of stillncss, the gap of silence we discussed in the previous chapter. Principle 1, *Be Present*, is like defibrillation. It helps us get into this gap.

Principle 2, *Become Aware*, teaches us to take advantage of this gap. It's a period of time when we can begin to listen, stay in the present moment, and start to understand what's really been happening around us. Although our patient is technically dead, we're going to bring him back to life again, a bit later. Right now, let's take advantage of this silence to learn what the health provider or rescuer does during this time.

As health providers, caring for a heart attack victim demands something of us: it demands that we, ourselves, become aware. If we freak out, get panicky, pass out from stress, or inadvertently stand in a puddle of water while firing an electrical current, we are at great risk of quickly becoming victims, too. Obviously, all of us lying around dead wouldn't do much for the long-term survival of our species. So what must health providers do while the victim is lying there, effectively dead?

Simply put, we have to check our own pulses first. We must make sure we're alive so that we can save the patient. We breathe. We relax and carefully check the scene for safety. We think. We *Become Aware*.

What do we need to become aware of? The best way to describe it is like staring at a picture. We have to see the whole picture. If part of the picture is obscured or hidden behind a piece of furniture, we can't see it for what it really is.

Within the context of our medical system, if we're going to find health, we must first become aware of a few details, some of which have become hidden from us for various reasons. We have to know how things work when viewing the bigger picture — not simply the current image that's been painted for us by wealthy corporate executives who would prefer that we see only their particular version.

The medical picture being painted for patients today is only part of the whole. Their perspective is like looking at a picture of the Mona

PRINCIPLE 2: BECOME AWARE | 73

Lisa that is cropped to show only her smile. This view is also only one perspective, and it would be very hard to determine what Mona Lisa looks like if we could only see the picture of her mouth. In order to truly shift our paradigm, we need to see the bigger picture. This chapter presents a new way of viewing four key stakeholders in healthcare: health insurance companies, lawyers, drug companies, and the government. It's simply a synopsis to provide you more information with which to formulate the next step along your journey toward health, instead of disease.

Often, these stakeholders don't provide patients with the big picture for two very simple reasons. First, if you as a patient didn't believe in the necessity of their products or services, you wouldn't be willing to help them continue to exist. Second, if you didn't believe they should exist, you would likely stop paying exorbitant amounts of money to them, and they wouldn't be able to earn big profits for their executives and investors.

Additionally, doctors often don't or won't tell you about the big picture for two key reasons. First, doctors are trained under the system that is controlled by these stakeholders, paid by the same system, and face potential legal and financial punishment by this system. The disease-oriented paradigm within which doctors are trained has made them afraid to tell you how it really works. Second, because doctors are trained extensively in disease, they spend 10 to 15 years inside their own disease boxes. They are often unable to see the big picture of embracing health first; rather, they fall back on their training, telling you that you must prevent disease as the means to becoming healthy. But recall, the absence of disease is merely the absence of disease and does not convey optimal health.

So, as we can begin to see, these four stakeholders operate to keep both patients and doctors in fear. You are afraid to get sick and die, so you pay for the promise that the healthcare system (i.e., the stakeholders) will keep you from getting sick or dying. But doctors cannot honor that promise. Doctors must preach only the message the system tells them to, because they are afraid of punishment, litigation, or financial loss. They recommend only treatments they've been trained to prescribe. In the end, both doctor and patient become victims of disease: the first unable to recommend health and the latter unable to find it.

74 | THE 7 PRINCIPLES OF HEALTH

To help us understand more about how our current medical system works, we'll need to examine a few statistics regarding how our healthcare system has "taken care" of us.

Health Statistics

In 2009, we spent $305 billion in the United States on preventable illnesses like heart disease, certain cancers, hypertension, diabetes, and high cholesterol.[5] The percent of overweight, obese, and extremely obese adults over the age of 20 years increased from 58.9 percent to 73.7 percent between the years 1988-94 and 2007-08.[6] In 1996, the percent of the adult population who had visited a physician to treat diabetes was 4.6, at a cost of $18.5 billion. By 2007, the percent of the adult population being treated for diabetes had doubled to 8.5, at a total cost of $40.8 billion.[7] The point of this brief synopsis is that we are sick and only getting sicker. We must find another way of doing things.

America spent $2.5 trillion on healthcare in 2009, a number that is projected to increase to $4.4 trillion by 2019.[8] In 1970, America spent only $75 billion on healthcare, but by 2006, this amount had increased to $2.1 trillion, a net increase of 2,711 percent.[9] Currently, these healthcare expenditures equate to a per person cost of $8,086, which is projected to increase to $13,387 by 2019.[10] A 2006 study by the McKinsey Global Institute showed that the United States spent $650 billion more on healthcare than other developed countries, and

---

[5]Total Expenses and Percent Distribution for Selected Conditions by Type of Service: United States, Medical Expenditure Panel Survey (MEPS), Agency for Healthcare Research and Quality. 2009

[6]Prevalence of Overweight, Obesity, and Extreme Obesity Among Adults: United States, Trends 1960 -1962 Through 2007-2008, National Center for Health Statistics, Health E-Stats. June 2010

[7]Trends in Use and Expenditures for Diabetes among Adults 18 and older, U.S. Civilian Non-institutionalized Population, 1996 and 2007, Statistical Brief #304, Medical Expenditure Panel Survey (MEPS), Agency for Healthcare Research and Quality. December 2010

[8]National Center for Health Statistics, United States, 2011: With Special Feature on Socioeconomic Status and Health. Hyattsville, MD. 2012

[9]Davidson, Steven M. *Still Broken: Understanding the U.S. Healthcare System.* Stanford University Press, Stanford, CA. 2010

[10]National Health Expenditures and Selected Economic Indicators, Levels and Annual Percent Change: Calendar Years 2004-2019, September 2010, Centers for Medicare and Medicaid Services, Office of the Actuary.

PRINCIPLE 2: BECOME AWARE | 75

a white paper by Thomson Reuters in October 2009 showed how $700 billion in waste could be eliminated annually from the American medical system.[11, 12] Between 2001 and 2009, health insurance premiums rose by 61.6 percent, employee contributions increased by 92.2 percent, and family premiums rose by 73.5 percent.[13] And to top it all off, health insurance companies posted profits of almost $265 billion during the worst years of America's Great Recession, 2008-10.[14]

The cost of Medicare increased from $311.3 billion in 2004 to $469.2 billion in 2008, and is projected to reach $977.8 billion by 2019. As a nation, we spent $234 billion on the top 10 therapeutic prescription drugs in 2010.[15] In 2004, *Bloomberg Businessweek* magazine reported that Merck & Co., makers of the prescription drug Vioxx® (which had just been pulled off the market due to dangerous side effects), had spent $3 billion a year on direct-to-consumer advertising for patented drugs (synthetic drugs which the pharmaceutical companies make and patent, thereby retaining exclusive rights to sell them).[16] Prior to that, we didn't really need a lot of pills to keep us healthy. After reviewing all of these health statistics, it's clear that we need to better understand whether we're paying for health or disease in the context of our current healthcare system.

It doesn't matter whether you understand all of the data just presented. The point is that even if you aren't currently sick or have not been diagnosed with a disease, you will be if you see a conventional medical doctor like me who's been trained to find disease in order to get paid and prescribe pills in order to fix you. And during your exam,

---

[11]Farrell, Diana et al. "Accounting for the cost of healthcare: A new look at why Americans spend more." McKinsey Global Institute. December 2008

[12]Kelley, Robert, VP. "Where can $700 billion in waste be cut annually from the U.S. healthcare system." Healthcare Analytics, Thomson Reuters. October 2009

[13]Changes in Premiums and Employee Contributions for Employer-Sponsored Health Insurance, Private Industry, 2001-2009, Medical Expenditure Panel Survey (MEPS), Statistical Brief #325, Agency for Healthcare Quality and Research. June 2011

[14]Potter, Wendell. *Deadly Spin: An Insurance Company Insider Speaks Out on How Corporate PR Is Killing Healthcare and Deceiving Americans.* Bloomsbury Press, New York. 2010

[15]Prescribed Drug Estimates: Medical Expenditure Panel Survey (MEPS), Agency for Healthcare Quality and Research. 2010

[16]"Lessons from the Vioxx Fiasco," *Bloomberg Businessweek* magazine, November 28, 2004. Accessed online at http://www.businessweek.com/stories/2004-11-28/lessons-from-the-vioxx-fiasco

your concerns will unavoidably shift toward preventing disease, rather than embracing health. Along with this shift, your thought system or mindset will then also be programmed to disease as opposed to health.

On your current health journey, you'll likely make significant financial investments toward disease prevention, some of which are actually bankrupting our fellow citizens. You may experience emotional stress about the cost of healthcare. This chronic worry and stress may lead to physical changes in your body. And before you know it, you'll be physically ill. The current healthcare system is designed to increase your potential to manifest real disease, either emotional, physical, or both.

What then happens is that we react to the events that led us there. We take on different attitudes — negative ones — that lead us into a vicious circle of emotions. When fear is the foundation of health, it leads to distraction and disempowerment, as we have discussed. It also leads to blame. Lawyers help us perpetuate the blame. They encourage you, the patient, to sue me, the doctor. But blame doesn't really help either of us. All it does is hold us hostage inside the vicious circle.

Blame may cause us to feel guilty and sabotage ourselves, externalizing our reasons for not becoming healthy, remaining disempowered, and failing to stand up to those who perpetuate the fear. Once we've sabotaged ourselves — whether financially, physically, or emotionally — we again become victims. We wait for things to change. We wait for someone else to change us. We accept messages, diagnoses, and paradigms we shouldn't accept. As victims, we become even more fearful of that inescapable thing we feared in the first place. The result is that this unfortunate collection of attitudes can lead us into a catastrophic cycle from which we may have tremendous trouble escaping.

That's the small, partially obscured picture.

A Bigger Picture

Our health is integrated into the five key components we discussed in the overview to this book: the physical, mental, emotional, financial, and spiritual aspects of our lives. When one or more of these components is out of balance, every aspect of our lives becomes unbalanced. Our financial stress regarding today's disease-focused medical system has contributed to our physical challenges, as evidenced by the health

PRINCIPLE 2: BECOME AWARE | 77

statistics above. Out of our own fear of disease, death, and dying, we have become victims of the modern medical system. And the stakeholders are all too willing to capitalize on those fundamental fears in order to generate still greater profits.

In the next section, we'll take a brief look at how each of these stakeholders has contributed to our choice to remain victims in search of health.

The Role of Stakeholders

HEALTH INSURANCE COMPANIES

"How can I help you?" the man behind the thick glass enclosure asks me.

It's a bright, sunny, postcard-perfect day in Arizona. I'm standing in the front lobby of the enormous Blue Cross and Blue Shield offices. "I'd like to speak with the CEO." My voice sounds clear and tight.

"Do you have an appointment?" he asks.

"No."

"Then you can't see him."

My jaw clamps hard. "I'm not leaving until I talk to someone," I reply. "Get me the head supervisor in charge of billing and claims."

"What's this about?"

"I want you guys to stop breeching my provider contract. You've kicked us out-of-network for no reason and now you're sending hundreds of thousands of dollars in payments directly to patients for our services. And tell your customer representatives to stop lying to my patients on the phone. You make it sound like it's our fault that you violated the contract."

I never did get to speak to the CEO. He was admitted to hospital that same day with a heart attack.

●

Prior to the managed care era, health insurance companies as we know them today didn't exist. The Health Maintenance Organization (HMO) Act was signed in 1973 by President Richard Nixon. With it, HMOs were put in place to control the cost of delivering health to Americans. This was (and still is) referred to as "administrative costs." This cost is

78 | THE 7 PRINCIPLES OF HEALTH

not for a doctor to provide his or her services. This is simply the cost of shuffling paper and advertising by health insurance companies to gain a larger market share. Administrative costs, despite all our technological advances and the push for electronic medical records, have increased from $2.8 billion in 1970 to $145.4 billion in 2006, a total increase of 5,093 percent.[17]

Private health insurance companies operate for-profit businesses. Some are listed on the stock exchanges as Fortune 500 and Fortune 1000 companies. They have investors and shareholders and they compete for investment money in the marketplace. They must consistently demonstrate that they are viable to investors and that they make healthy profits; if they don't, investors will shift their money to other more viable companies. Health insurance companies continue to exist because they can reliably show their investors that they make healthy profits.

How does a health insurance company show profits when it does not sell any products? If a company doesn't sell a product, it usually sells a service. In this case, health insurance companies sell the service of administering the cost of the healthcare system. How do health insurance companies administer the cost of healthcare services and still show profits? There are only two other entities left in the equation: you, as their beneficiary, and I, as the doctor or provider of actual health services. Basically, the health insurance company asks you to sign up for their insurance, takes your money, and puts it in their own pocket, via the bank. In the meantime, the insurance company promises that when you need help with your disease, it will pay for the cost of your care. When you come to me for health services, you don't pay directly. I have to negotiate a contract with the health insurance company in order to get paid.

But the health insurance company still needs to post profits in the middle of a healthcare crisis, and it can only get its money from you or from me. So what does it do? It charges you more money for the promise of healthcare at some future date, effectively increasing your insurance premiums and deductibles. It also pays me less for my professional services, thereby decreasing reimbursement to doctors.

---

[17]Davidson, *Still Broken*.

PRINCIPLE 2: BECOME AWARE | 79

That way it keeps more money for itself so it can prove to its investors that it makes a lot of money on the stock exchange. The more money the health insurance company keeps in its bank account, the greater its profits.

So what happens when the cost of technology rises, the population ages, and people's ever-expanding illnesses require more expensive services? The health insurance company must pay for health services, which decreases their profits. But they really love to make a profit, don't they? So what can they do to try and keep their profit margins high? You already know the answer.

They have three options:

1. They can charge you more and more for health insurance.
2. They can decrease payments to me, a doctor.
3. They can deny you services if you get very sick and require treatment.

If they do all three, they will keep even more money and be able to show their investors a sizeable profit for that year.

Why does the cost of health insurance keep rising when these companies continue to post profits? Health insurance executives say that the cost of the delivery of services (i.e., the administrative cost) is increasing. They say that they must pay doctors more money, and that technology costs are increasing these days. They tell us that this is what it costs to keep us healthy because as we age, we are getting sicker. But in reality, we are not healthy! Take a look at the statistics again. You've been paying them to help with your health, but the money you've spent has gone into disease, as witnessed by the epidemics of our modern era!

The only explanation, then, is that the *administrative cost* is increasing. But how can that be? These companies were put in place to control administrative cost! That doesn't make any sense, does it? The cost that you and I pay to control costs is escalating beyond belief. This must mean the amount they need to take in to *post a profit* is what's skyrocketing. In other words, the earnings health insurance companies need in order to show consistent profits correlate almost directly to the increases in your health insurance payments (e.g., premiums, deductibles, co-payments, co-insurance, etc.) and the decreases in payouts to doctors in the form of reimbursements.

80 | THE 7 PRINCIPLES OF HEALTH

During the last five years of the worst healthcare crisis in the United States, United Health Group highlighted a revenue increase of $7 billion in its 2010 earnings report, boasting that it "achieved business growth across each of its reporting segments."[18] United Health Group is not the only private sector company operating this way. They all do, which is why they are called health *insurance* companies and not *healthcare* companies. We have blindly interpreted their messages to mean that they will care for our health. They do no such thing.

How are they able to do this? In the end, it all boils down to fear. The sicker you are, the more afraid you become, and the more afraid you become, the more you are willing to pay them for the promise that they will care for you in the future, when you become even sicker still. They must keep you in fear so that you'll keep paying.

How do they keep you afraid? Health insurance companies have trained you to think that you need them to stay healthy. They assure you that they will pay when you get sick. And so you pay them your hard-earned money, money that could have gone into keeping you healthy today but instead is now going toward some speculative future illness that may or may not ever occur. As long as you continue to funnel your money toward some future date and future sickness, forgetting to take steps to keep yourself healthy now, you are all but guaranteed to get sicker and eventually require their services.

What do you think they'll say at that future date, when many, many more people are sick and require procedures such as bypass surgeries, cancer treatments, transplants, joint replacements, and dialysis? You guessed it! They are likely to deny you services for healthcare. The irony is these "medical" issues are largely preventable, degenerative, inflammatory diseases. If we take the steps toward practicing health now and use our money to help us stay well, we may not require such extensive disease-focused procedures in the future.

Human nature seems fundamentally afraid of disease and death. As a result, we continue to believe that health insurance companies are a necessary component of healthcare in America. We continue to blindly pay and pay, victims in a bizarre health insurance drama that's playing out before our eyes.

---

[18]United Health Group Annual Report 2010. Accessed online at: http://www.unitedhealthgroup.com/2010-annual-report.

PRINCIPLE 2: BECOME AWARE | 81

Not only are we victims of health insurance, but we are victims of our own fears. And it's these fears that have driven us to pay someone else to alleviate them. But no matter how much we pay, no one else out there can protect us from disease and death. When greed and profit become intertwined with a false promise like this, fear must be continuously perpetuated or the money train filled with profits will screech to a halt. As a result, sickness *must* be the default.

Remove the fear of death and disease, and people will live for health. They will act for health. They will practice health, and they will manifest health in their bodies, minds, emotions, spirits, and bank accounts. All five components of total health — not disease — will fall into balance. And that would eradicate the need for health insurance companies entirely.

YOUR INVITATION TO PRACTICE HEALTH

You are welcome to visit health-conscious.org, where you can learn more about how much your own health insurance has really cost you. The Personal Health Insurance Cost Calculator is a quick reference tool that will enable you to calculate how much you've actually spent over the last five years on healthcare. There's not much work involved on your part. It's simply a tool designed to help you become aware of whether the trade off you're making by paying health insurance out of a fear of disease is worth it, or if the money might be better spent on taking care of your health today.

LAWYERS

Lawyers' jobs are to protect individual rights — mostly their own. America was largely founded on individual rights, and the words "I'll sue you!" have become an inherent component of that philosophy. As with many other aspects of life, when it comes to medicine, someone must be to blame.

But what is the price of blame? Most people don't understand that the cost of an individual's right to sue over a problem with healthcare service is directly transferred to every person in the country who

82 | THE 7 PRINCIPLES OF HEALTH

pays for healthcare. Individuals who consider their right to sue integral to the delivery of healthcare should not complain that they can't afford the high cost of health insurance anymore. All those lawsuits are directly related to how much every one of us pays.

How does the cost of the individual right to sue get transferred to personal healthcare expenses? Doctors, the ones people blame for bad outcomes in the delivery of healthcare services, protect themselves against a patient's option to sue with a tool called malpractice insurance. In order to defend themselves against potential lawsuits, individual doctors purchase malpractice insurance. In addition to protecting themselves with insurance, physicians also try to protect themselves in the way they deliver services.

Let's take a look at an emergency room doctor who, due to the nature of her practice, has a greater risk of getting sued. This is not because she is a bad doctor or wants to cause harm, but because of the high risk inherent in emergency situations. Not everyone survives, regardless of how skilled the doctor is. Such is life. People die, as we have noted earlier. Death is something we must all learn to accept.

But because our culture has a particularly difficult time with death, the emergency room doctor will order as many tests as possible, dig around for as many unusual diseases as possible, and send the patient for as many procedures as possible before she releases him or her to go home. This is known as defensive medicine. The doctor is first taking as many steps as she can to defend herself against lawyers, providing her patient with healthcare inside this medical system is a seemingly distant second.

But no matter how many tests she orders or how many procedures she performs as an experienced doctor, life can take unexpected turns. Complications arise. Doctors rely on statistics in their practice; they accept that there is a certain level of complication inherent in every pill dispensed, every test ordered, every procedure performed, and every person treated. Again, this is not because they are bad doctors, but because they are human, and life is what it is. There are no guarantees.

Lawyers cannot allow that doctors are human if they are to advocate for your right to sue and your right to blame someone for your

PRINCIPLE 2: BECOME AWARE | 83

hurt. Money motivates them to find doctors' flaws and failings. Multiply the defensive practice of medicine by thousands of doctors and millions of patient visits in any place that delivers healthcare services (e.g., clinics, doctors' offices, emergency rooms, outpatient surgery centers, hospitals, imaging centers, etc.) and we add another layer to our healthcare crisis. The estimated cost of defensive medicine in America is between $650 and $850 billion annually.[19] The total dollars paid in malpractice claims was $3.177 billion in 2011.[20] Only 20 percen of the total settlement goes to the patient (plaintiff); 80 percent goes to lawyers.

While the media in the United States tends to focus on multimillion dollar awards, the average settlement was actually smaller than in Canada and the United Kingdom in 2001.[21] Through it all, we remain victims, utterly disempowered and distracted by false promises. And we incorporate an attitude of blame to further wedge a gap between patient and doctor — a toxic divide in a relationship that's supposed to be founded on health and healing.

DRUG COMPANIES

Most people today agree that they would rather not take a pill. They have come to understand that synthetic pills have helped us with certain issues, but they come with a risk — sometimes many, many risks. Over time, people have come to understand that not all things can be fixed with a pill and that, more often than not, the addition of drugs for the treatment of one condition often leads to side effects and complications that affect other bodily systems.

Half a century ago, penicillin was touted as the cure-all for almost everything. Many people who grew up during the penicillin era now go to see their doctors with a cold and ask for a "shot." That shot used to be penicillin. Colds however, are the result of various viruses which,

---

[19] A costly defense — Physicians sound off on the high price of defensive medicine, Jackson Healthcare and Gallop Surveys. October 2009

[20] The Henry Kaiser Family Foundation, State Health Facts. Accessed online at http://www.statehealthfacts.org

[21] Anderson, Gerard F. et. al. Health Spending in the United States and the Rest of the Industrialized World. Health Affairs. July 2005. Accessed online at http://content.healthaffairs.org/content/24/4/903. full#sec-7

84 | THE 7 PRINCIPLES OF HEALTH

though annoying to us, are rarely life threatening. And viruses do not respond to antibiotics like penicillin because antibiotics only treat bacterial infections. What has happened is that penicillin has been so overused that the bacteria it was originally meant to treat have mutated and changed their protective mechanisms. They have become largely resistant to penicillin, which means that penicillin is no longer as effective as it used to be.

Today, we're facing bacteria for which we have no effective medication. This has led to dramatic reports in the news media about things like "flesh-eating" bacteria. What this really means is that our overuse of medications in the past has created a new race of bugs for which we no longer have cures. In addition, our immune systems have weakened through the overuse of drugs. Because we never allowed ourselves to fully heal, our systems are no longer strong enough to defend against these common organisms.

Another problem has arisen from the drug industry itself. Pharmaceutical companies are in business to make money, which they do with patented drugs. What's the best way to sell a drug? Tell patients they need it. An even better way to sell drugs is to tell patients the one with the ® trademark is the best one to take. A better way yet is to tell someone they will get sick and die if they don't take your drug — the one you've patented and protected.

Perhaps the most brilliant way to sell a drug is to train a health professional who prescribes drugs to convince their sick and dying patients that using your patented drug is the only alternative for their healing.

●

Candy has a sore throat today. She looks miserable sitting on the exam table. "Were your tests negative for strep throat?"[22] I ask Candy.

"Yes."

"Then why did your doctor give you antibiotics? Your illness isn't bacterial — it's a virus. Antibiotics don't work on viruses, and your test was negative. It doesn't make sense to give you a drug your body doesn't need."

"They told me to take it anyway, just because."

---

[22]Strep throat occurs when streptococci bacteria infect the throat; it is treatable with antibiotics.

PRINCIPLE 2: BECOME AWARE | 85

In 2005, the FDA approved 80 new medications. It also recalled 401 prescription drugs and 101 over-the-counter drugs the same year.[23] A large percentage of drugs approved by the FDA are pulled off the market due to harmful side effects. Anyone who cites FDA approval as "scientifically proven" should ask themselves if they want to be the person in that class-action lawsuit who will die in six months from irreversible heart disease after using an FDA-approved drug that was "proven" safe.

Drug companies must create disease; it is the foundation of their existence. When so much money is at stake, health is just not an option. They use doctors' narrow scope of training to convince them that prescription drugs are the only options to offer their patients, and because of their extensive training in disease and its cures, doctors are unable to see any other choices.

In order for drug companies to keep making money from our inability to find true health, both doctor and patient must remain their victims.

GOVERNMENT

Between 1960 and 1980, the cost of Medicare doubled every four years. In 2002, the cost was $256 billion; by 2007 the cost had risen to $440 billion; and in 2008 the cost had reached $599 billion.[24] The Medicare program is expected to go bankrupt by 2019 — possibly sooner — as of the time of this writing.

Where's all this money supposed to come from? It's supposed to come from us, the taxpayers. The problem is that the younger generations (ages 19 to 65) are footing the bill for those who actually use these healthcare services. In other words, approximately 80 percent or more of the population (ages 19 to 65) is paying for the less than 20 percent (ages 65+) who use expensive healthcare services. Our

---

[23]Center for Drug Evaluation and Research, Report to the Nation 2005, U.S. Department of Health and Human Services, Food and Drug Administration, Center for Drug Evaluation and Research.

[24]National Health Expenditures and Selected Economic Indicators, Levels and Annual Percent Change: Calendar Years 2004-2019, Centers for Medicare and Medicaid Services, Office of the Actuary. September 2010

86 | THE 7 PRINCIPLES OF HEALTH

younger generations are squandering their hard-earned money to pay for this monstrous amount of disease and profit, effectively guaranteeing that they will get sick in the future because they cannot afford to take good care of themselves now.

The other problem is that our younger generation is also aging. We all grow older as human beings. Right now, the ratio of people younger than 65 years is 0.7 to 2.5 people older than 65. By 2019, there will be 0.4 people younger than 65 to 3.2 people older than 65. Who's going to pay the $4.4 trillion bill when all of those people who are currently young become sick and old because they used the majority of their paychecks to pay for today's elderly, sick, and dying?

If someone were to ask you how you would want to spend your old age — lying on a hospital bed hooked to machines, deathly ill but surviving two extra months on chemotherapy, or enjoying a high quality of life, playing your favorite sport — how would you answer?

Our medical system has developed phenomenal advancements in technology which, combined with doctors' terrific egos, have convinced many of us that we can cheat death. This has led to the belief that death is no longer acceptable. So we pump life into the dying process in the form of expensive healthcare treatments. The dying process has become sterilized and medicalized to the point where a person's dignity and self-respect is the very last consideration. As physicians, we force conditions on others which we, ourselves, would never tolerate. Why do we insist on keeping our loved ones alive at all costs? Is it simply for the sake of satisfying our own egos?

This next generation — you and I — are riddled with devastating, preventable diseases: heart disease, hypertension, type 2 diabetes, high cholesterol, and many types of cancers. Subsequently, we will not live as long as our parents who did not grow up with Medicare, government programs, or privatized health insurance. Though they've been increasing up until today, our future life spans will shorten. No amount of money we spend now on those who are long past dying will help us live healthy lives in the future, and any fixes offered to us will be unaffordable.

In order to pay for its existence, and to perpetuate the myth of immortality to the constituents of those running for political office, the government must continue to promise that health is just around the corner, as long as we all keep our heads down and keep paying. And to maintain the status quo, if we dare to question, there'll be plenty of punishment for both patients and doctors — things like mandatory health insurance and reductions in reimbursements for not making patients "healthy" inside a broken system.

DOCTORS

Throughout the centuries, the medical profession has always maintained an air of mystery. From shamans to witch doctors to snake oil salesmen to modern-day physicians, the layperson has never been completely comfortable with doctor types. Perhaps it's because their knowledge of life and death, or the mystery of our own bodies, has led people to believe that doctors are somehow "in the know." People who are "in the know" can be intimidating to others, especially if they know how to save us from death!

So doctors are often viewed as authority figures, meaning they tell people what to do and how to do it. They tell people how to heal and how to save their lives because they *know*. To question a doctor is to question the authority of one who understands life and death. Patients are expected *not* to question; they are expected to follow all their doctors' orders.

This attitude is a paternalistic way of practicing medicine. The doctor becomes something of a father or parent figure, as he or she always knows what's best for you. The patient then plays the role of the child and is not allowed to think, act, or choose for themselves.

But the origin of the word doctor comes from the Latin *docēre*, which means "to teach." This puts patients and doctors into very different roles; the relationship becomes one of teacher and student, rather than parent and child. The student comes to learn from the teacher. The student can then choose to use the knowledge he or she has learned to make his or her own decisions.

Reflect on some of your encounters with physicians in our modern medical system. Have your visits been educational, more like the teacher and student, or are they more like a parent would act toward a disobedient child? Have your doctors taken time to explain things well and teach you about the many different options available, including those from complementary and alternative practices? Have they supported you in the choices you make, even if those choices were contrary to their own advice?

88 | THE 7 PRINCIPLES OF HEALTH

Unfortunately, many people report that they have been told which prescriptions to take, which tests to have performed, and which lifestyle changes to make. They are not advised, supported, or coached about other options. A typical exam with a doctor these days lasts about seven minutes. Most doctors do not — and cannot — take the time to talk about the many different aspects of health with their patients, including the psychological, emotional, or spiritual components.

Many patients report that their encounters with allopathic, or conventional, doctors are not as comprehensive as they would like. Rather, their conversations are very disease focused: "How can we correct your high cholesterol?" or "When will we test for diabetes?" rather than "How can we make you feel great by addressing your nutrition, exercise, and emotional state?" The experience of doctor and patient today is not one of teacher and student but one of authoritarian command.

This authoritarian attitude continues to be perpetuated in Western medicine. Doctors typically use words like, "Why didn't you take your medication?" or "I told you to lose weight and exercise." A sense of fear may then arise within the patient, as though they have done something wrong or displeased their doctors. Add this to an authoritarian attitude around the mystery of life and death, and it becomes extremely difficult and intimidating to understand which choices you can or should make about the disease label your doctor has given you. You may not even be able to pronounce the name of the illness! Without intention, we doctors have intensified your sense of fear about your disease. As a result, you may be more likely to follow our instructions than question or refute our "authority" in order to make choices for yourself.

Do doctors intend to create fear or disempower their patients? Of course not! Then why do they do it? In order to answer that question, we need to examine the way doctors are trained.

America values specialists, borne out by the fact that there are more than three specialists for every general practitioner in America.[25] Specialists are trained for three to six years after graduating in their area of specialization. They focus on one very detailed aspect of the human body. They have metaphorically glued their eyes to the microscope and

---

[25]National Center for Health Statistics, Health, United States, Hyattsville, MD: NCHS. 2007

have broken you apart into your mechanical parts. And you, as the patient, have demanded specialists. You want the expert to check your heart, your skin, your eyes, your hair, and your toenails. The problem is that these specialists have been so highly trained in one very specific area of the body that they cannot put you back together. They do not know how to step back and integrate you into the big picture of health. Nor do they care to do so, as they are typically more interested in their medicine specialty than in your overall health. Specialists expect the primary care doctor to do that.

The emerging problem is that there is now a serious shortage of primary care providers, leaving you in the hands of specialists to try and care for your overall health. You then get bounced back and forth between many different doctors, none of whom really want to put you back together again into an integrated, whole person, because that's not what they have been trained to do. The consequence is that your medical care has become highly fragmented. Slip that into the context of a broken medical system, and we can see why many patients come home with a list of 20 different pills, each prescribed by a different doctor who has not considered the person as an integrated, living system.

Is it any wonder we can no longer put ourselves back together under this type of a medical system to become whole and healthy? The attempt is almost futile. There seems to be no one out there who is approaching health from a new perspective, using a different way of thinking to shift the paradigm.

Somehow, the strength to heal is going to have to come from somewhere deep inside you. You are going to have to stop the distraction that's been keeping you from becoming aware of what's really happening in medicine today. You must empower yourself, releasing your fears, distraction, and victimization, and find health by shifting toward a new paradigm for your future.

Disease Currency

In an earlier chapter, we discussed The Current Health Paradigm and examined the many different words used to describe our current health system. Now that you've become aware of a different perspective, let's try a brief exercise. The Current Health Paradigm has been

90 | THE 7 PRINCIPLES OF HEALTH

reproduced here. Take a moment to circle the words which resonate with you when you consider our healthcare system.

Current Health Paradigm

Quick Fix	Rapid cures, band-aid solutions, band-aid cures
Fragmentation	Broken apart, disjointed, disconnected, unconnected, redundant, separated into pieces or subcomponents
Individualism	Concerned with the person as individual vs. the common, group, or collective interest; egoism; placing priority on individuals first, and not the collective; lack of sharing; concern with the self over others; prioritizing "me" first
Cure	Eliminate, correct, restore, get rid of, fix
Disease Orientation	Focusing on a disordered or non-functioning part, structure, or system; targeting study, prevention, and cure toward the abnormal or sickened component of the human body
Mechanization	Separating the whole into its interrelated parts; Newtonian physics; mechanistic; the sum of a body's parts equates to the whole when put together; focusing on individual parts instead of complex, integrated systems; using cause and effect instead of integrated functions
Polarization	At opposite ends of the spectrum; separated or divided; apart (EXAMPLES: conventional vs. complementary/alternative; East vs. West; allopathic vs. holistic; traditional vs. natural medicine)
Victimization	Disempowerment; lack of choice; doing things as you've been told; having things done to you against your will; lack of will power

PRINCIPLE 2: BECOME AWARE | 91

Paternalism	Parent/child relationship comprised of orders, rules, dictates, management, or governance with punishment and/or reward; physician/doctor-centered models in medicine
Mandates	Dictates; orders; being told what to do; punishment as a consequence; bureaucracy; outside party involvement; command or demand to act in a particular way
Blame	To hold someone else responsible; lack of responsibility or accountability; to find fault in someone or something else
Judgment	Determination; conclusion; authoritative opinion; assessment or decision
Myopic Perspective	Narrow-sighted; tunnel-visioned; near-sighted; close-minded; narrow-minded; small picture view vs. big picture view; short-sighted
Unconsciousness	Unaware; not perceived at the level of awareness; not brought into one's conscious mindset or thinking

Are these words necessarily our reality? Or could they just be words which currently describe our health and health system? Could we begin to choose different words and use their meaning to define a different reality for ourselves? Reproduced here is The New Health Paradigm and the words associated with it.

New Health Paradigm

Long Term	Longevity (as in long life); for a long period of time; long-lasting; far-reaching; for the longest time possible; for life or lifelong
Whole	Undivided; integrated; all parts connected; together; collective; entire person; integral; unbroken; intact; complete
Collective	Forming a whole; combined; characteristics of a group of individuals taken together (as in society); synergistic; concerned with the group instead of the individual; functioning as a unit as opposed to separate pieces; a sum of parts

92 | THE 7 PRINCIPLES OF HEALTH

Healing	Bring to optimal health; make functional again; to restore to completeness or become whole again
Health	A general condition of the whole; a focus on achieving optimal wellness or optimal function in many aspects of life (EXAMPLES: mental, emotional, physical, social, environmental, financial, etc.); relieving the presence of dis-ease (lack of ease); assisting the body to rid itself of disease and return to a state of vigor, energy, or vitality
Energetic System	Multidimensional; Einsteinian physics; integration; inseparability; quantum theories; the whole is more than the sum of its parts; a way of viewing things as complex systems, rather than mechanical parts; viewing things as integrated functions rather than separable parts
Balance	Bringing together opposing sides equally; giving equal weight to different sides; a state of equilibrium; adjusting the portions symmetrically; avoiding excesses of one thing; moderation
Empowerment	Giving power; choice; authority; operating by personal will; enablement; will power; self-authority; making your own decisions; having the will or authority to decide
Guide or Teacher	Teacher/student relationships; assist in another's decision making; help, accompany; provide knowledge; instruct; lead; collaborate; work together; share
Collaboration	Supporting or working with one another; cooperation; working together; give and take; shared-decision making
Accountability	Responsibility; holding the self responsible; obligation to oneself; self-drive; answerability to the self
Nonjudgment	Without critical assessment or opinion; objective; without criticizing; without inference; without critical opinion
Clear Vision	Seeing things clearly, as in perception; 20/20; state of being transparent; freedom from indistinctness or ambiguity
Consciousness	State of awareness; knowing; being aware; participating in all sensations, perceptions, or activities; full presence

PRINCIPLE 2: BECOME AWARE | 93

What if we were to begin with these words as our fundamental belief system? What if we were then to create a reality that began with these words foremost in our minds? As we have mentioned, everything in life is created twice, first in our minds and then manifest in our world. These words are simply that — *words*. They are not reality. They are what we call scripts or messages or programs, and the ones from the first table currently make up our belief system surrounding health and healthcare, as individuals and as a collective nation. What if we were to rescript or reprogram our messages, beginning with words like "integrated" or "health" first, and then proceeded to create a different reality based on these new messages?

I invite you to read the following sentences aloud and listen to some of the messages we hear every day:

- "You have two, maybe three, weeks to live."
- "What are you going to do without insurance?! You'll die!"
- "How am I going to pay for my kid's healthcare? How am I going to afford all this for my family?"
- "Just give me the pill, Doc."
- "Fix me, Doc. I don't have time for this."
- "Can you change this diagnosis to something different? My insurance won't cover this."
- "Why didn't you come for your checkups? What if you have a disease?"
- "If you don't follow my advice to have a hysterectomy, you'll hurt my feelings as your doctor."
- "My doctor says that I have to _____."
- "This disease is a death sentence. I can't do anything about it."
- "Maybe it's the coffee that's keeping me from getting better."
- "My sugar's is high because I had a donut this morning. Normally, it's very low."

These sentences are a collection of Western society's disease currency. Some of them may not seem all that strange to you. In fact, they might sound so normal that you're asking what's wrong with them. But in our new health paradigm, we can take a look at the underlying messages and attitudes that we convey with these sentences.

94 | THE 7 PRINCIPLES OF HEALTH

- **Disease/Doctor-Centric Paternalism:** "You have two, maybe three weeks to live."
- **Fear/Victimization:** "What are you going to do without insurance? You'll die."
- **Fear/Disempowerment:** "How am I going to pay for my kid's healthcare? How am I going to afford all this for my family?"
- **Fix/Quick Fix/Cure:** "Just give me the pill, Doc" and "Fix me, Doc, I don't have time for this."
- **Disease/Mandate/Punishment:** "Can you change this diagnosis to something different? My insurance won't cover this."
- **Fear/Disempowerment/Paternalism:** "Why didn't you come for your checkups? What if you have a disease?"
- **Paternalism/Disease/Victimization:** "If you don't get a hysterectomy, you'll hurt my feelings as your doctor."
- **Paternalism/Victimization/Disempowerment:** "My doctor says that I have to _____."
- **Blame/Fear/Disease/Disempowerment/Victimization:** "This disease is a death sentence. I can't do anything about it."
- **Blame/Disease/Cure:** "Maybe it's the coffee that's keeping me from getting better."
- **Blame/Disease/Victimization:** "My sugar's is high because I had a donut this morning. Normally, it's very low."

You might be able to match even more words from The Current Health Paradigm with these very real sentences I hear every day in my practice, but I'm sure you get the idea. We all need to begin with a new messaging system, new programming from which to focus, pursue, and live in optimal health.

●

Brittney is a personal trainer. She told me about a friend of hers who was recently diagnosed with breast cancer.

"I tried to give her a book for her birthday, *The Cure*, by Timothy Brantley," she said. "Maybe you've heard of it. He's a naturopath who talks about nutrition. My friend took it for a while, but then she gave it back."

"Why?" I asked, truly curious.

Brittney laughed. "She said it 'just wasn't for her.' She decided to go the medical route, with surgery, chemotherapy and radiation," she explained, shaking her head. "The book is about eating high quality food. I can't believe she thinks chemotherapy alone is going to help her!"

●

My financial advisor recently told me: "Greed and power know no boundaries." When profit is at the root of healthcare delivery systems, the outcome required — the outcome demanded — is disease, not health. There is no middle ground. And beware: those in control will stop at nothing to keep it that way.

YOUR INVITATION TO PRACTICE HEALTH

Here are a few questions to consider, related to your place in The Current Health Paradigm.

1. Make a short list of your diagnosed diseases or problems (emotional or physical). Try and be as honest with yourself as possible. If you don't have anything to put on your list, are you overweight or stressed out? If you still don't have anything to write down, are you worried about any genetic conditions you may inherit in the future?

   _____

   _____

2. Write down how you feel about each of those diagnoses. For example, if you have hypertension, write about how you think you may be different from someone who does not have hypertension.

   _____

   _____

96 | THE 7 PRINCIPLES OF HEALTH

3. Are you worried about any complications from your disease? For example, with hypertension, are you worried that it will cause a stroke?

_____

_____

4. What have you been told by your family, friends, and health professionals about your diagnosis?

_____

_____

5. Write down what your health insurance company has said or done about your diagnosis. Have you admitted to your health insurance provider that you have been diagnosed with a medical condition? Why or why not?

_____

_____

6. Are you afraid or worried about anything else regarding your health? Why or why not?

_____

_____

7. Do you feel that you have the power to change your future? Why or why not?

_____

_____

PRINCIPLE 2: BECOME AWARE | 97

8. Do you feel that someone (the government, health insurance, lawyers, or pharmaceutical companies) is going to improve our health as citizens of this country? Do you think this improvement will take place in your lifetime? What state of healthcare do you think you will be leaving behind for your children? Why do you feel this way? Try and support your answers with solid reasoning.

_____

_____

_____

_____

CHAPTER FIVE

Principle 3
Be Health

"Disease is cured by the body itself,
not by doctors or remedies."

— John Harvey Kellogg, M.D. *(1852-1943)*
American physician and creator
of the Corn Flakes® breakfast cereal

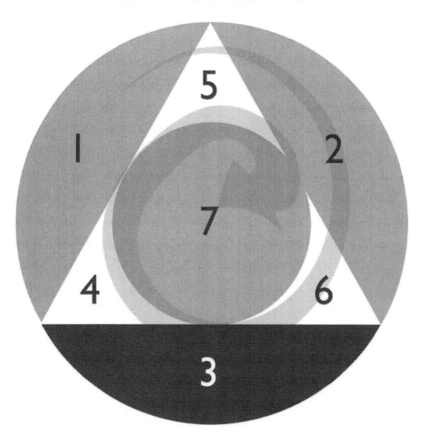

Our Thought Environment

In the last chapter, we learned a little about our healthcare system and the current way we view health, both as doctors and as patients. My hope is that seeing things from a different perspective will enable us to begin thinking about the next steps we might take in making our own health choices.

Principle 3, *Be Health*, introduces us to the way our thoughts can affect our health. The field of brain-mapping in neuroscience seeks to advance the understanding between the structure of our brains and the way we function. Originally studied in the 1930s by famous neurosurgeon Dr. Wilder Penfield, brain-mapping is now funded and researched by many large organizations, including the National Institutes of Health and the National Science Foundation. Advanced technology such as MRI (magnetic resonance imaging), MEG (magnetoencephalography), and PET (positron emission tomography) are often used to correlate the physical processes which underlie human sensation, awareness, and cognition. The results are applied to intervention and treatment in the areas of neurosurgery and psychiatry.

> *"You may not be what you think you are, but what you think, you are."*
>
> **— Jim Clark**

The field of neurolinguistic programming (NLP) is more controversial and seems to have morphed from its foundations in academic research into business and motivational success models. It generally refers to the connection between our brain, our language, and our subsequent behavior. Because the science behind NLP is more subjective (i.e., based on psychological and counseling techniques rather than scientific instrumentation), heated debate between the scientific community and the business community continues today. Nevertheless, highly successful motivational speakers like Anthony Robbins credit our ability to transform our lives to techniques like NLP.

The difference between brain-mapping and NLP seems to lie in the paradigm from which we operate. For example, as we've discussed so far, medicine currently uses a "fix it after it's broken" viewpoint. The study of brain-mapping largely delves into disease states, such as

100 | THE 7 PRINCIPLES OF HEALTH

Parkinson's, autism, and other cognitive disorders, seeking to find ways to cure or fix them. Neurolinguistic programming seems to work in a proactive way and is, perhaps, the reason many are attracted to its precepts. The statement, "You are what you think you are," holds true in this context. If you believe it, you can become it.

With this brief examination of these two divergent fields, the question ultimately remains with you, again. Which paradigm do you choose? While we cannot always explain every detail in disease and medicine at this juncture in our evolution, is it necessary to wait for those particular answers before we seek to change our health?

Let's take a look at body image, as an example. People map their thoughts to a certain perceived body image. The way they think they look may not necessarily match their actual height and weight measurements. A morbidly obese man might have recently lost more than 100 pounds. But until he sees himself as a thinner person, he may move, act, and think of himself exactly as he was before he lost the weight. He may walk with a heavy step that makes a casual observer who has never met him before think he "looks" much heavier than he actually is. What about a heavyset woman who perceives herself as light and graceful? Her elegant movements originate from the confident way she views her own body, regardless of what others may think and regardless of her actual measurements. We, as observers, may comment that she appears to be "comfortable in her own skin."

Let's go back to the preprogrammed sentences from the medical field that we used as examples in the last chapter. "You need to remember that you are sick" or "You have to do _____ or you will contract _____." We can put almost any action or disease into these blanks and hear the engrained messages of our current health paradigm.

But what if we each began with a message that read something like this: "In this moment, I am healthy. I feel good, regardless of this disease challenge, I may have. Let me take a look at some areas where I can choose differently in order to optimize my health. How might I eat differently? How might I think differently? What career would reduce the stress in my life and lead to a physical change in my blood pressure?" These are some extensive behavioral approaches any individual can undertake to shape a treatment plan that is founded in health first,

PRINCIPLE 3: BE HEALTH | 101

and not the specific management or prevention of disease. By focusing first on health and then seeking to correct a few lifestyle factors, rather than focusing first on drugs to correct the disease, the disease is concurrently corrected.

Lance Armstrong, the famous Tour de France cyclist, faced testicular cancer during his career. He says of his journey, "Through my illness, I learned rejection. I was written off. That was the moment I thought, 'Okay, game on. No prisoners. Everybody's going down.'" What do you think would have happened if he'd programmed his thoughts to the following phrases? "I'm sick. I'm a loser. My disease is a death sentence." Many of us steeped in The Current Health Paradigm might say these exact words if we were facing such a diagnosis. *(Please note, mention of Armstrong is not an endorsement. Though his Tour de France wins have been discredited due to the infamous doping scandal, Armstrong's cancer recovery still stands as a triumphant example of what is possible.)*

Cancer certainly is a very devastating diagnosis and can be a death sentence for some. But if we buy into this belief from the start, before we've actually died, and we begin to think we're going to die while we're still living, what do you think will happen to us physically? Our bodies will respond to our thought environment. Whether or not you need neuroscience to explain this, using advanced technology, the conclusion seems to be self-evident. Our outcomes depend on how we train our mind.

As we've become aware, the messages embedded in today's healthcare system contain a great deal of negative programming. And we've bought into much of them. There's also a tremendous amount of paradoxical or inconsistent messaging. For example, health insurance companies reimburse doctors for fixing disease, not preventing it or optimizing a patient's health. But they simultaneously profess to offer many programs for wellness and prevention. Yet Medicare has cut back payments to practitioners who begin with health and wellness in mind. For example, chiropractors, massage therapists, nutritionists, acupuncturists, and many other wellness providers are not covered by Medicare options, although our country is paying a tremendous amount for those supposed "health" benefits.

Additionally, pharmaceutical companies have run out of new antibiotic drugs to patent, so they're targeting cancer treatments as

102 | THE 7 PRINCIPLES OF HEALTH

potentially profitable. Do you think they want you to actually prevent cancer by eating right, exercising, and living a stress-free life when they'll only make their tremendous profits by treating you with expensive chemotherapeutic agents? Your diagnosis of cancer is worth billions to these companies, as we have seen by the advertising dollars spent on drugs in the previous chapter.

When we come to understand more about Principle 3, *Be Health*, perhaps long before we've manifested health by current medical definitions, we begin to understand that we are already "health" — right here and right now. We have the choice and the power to reprogram our thoughts and minds to believe that. We don't have to accept disease as our starting point or embrace the belief that in order to find health, we must first prevent disease. It makes no sense to seek health that way. The definition of health is not the absence of disease; it is the embodiment of optimal health practice and balance in every aspect of our lives, regardless of any labels the doctor may have saddled us with.

Here's an example. Our front desk staff member is 23 years old. She's five foot four and weighs 160 pounds. She runs out to McDonald's or Wendy's or gets fast-food Mexican cuisine for lunch every day. She drinks three to six cans of Coke during her shift and takes a smoke break every two hours. Would you say she's healthy? Technically, using the perspective of The Current Health Paradigm, she is healthy. But do her habits reflect health and balance?

Now compare this young lady to Allison, who had metastatic breast cancer. Which of the two is considered healthy, according to The New Health Paradigm? In this case, the definition of health is not indicated by writing "metastatic breast cancer" on paper, but the fact that all components of total health are in complete balance. Recall that *The 5 Components of Total Health* include our physical, emotional, mental/cognitive, spiritual, and financial components.

In order to program or rescript our own minds, to change the way we think regardless of the messages we hear in the medical community, we must always *Be Health* first. This is tough, I admit. Don't forget, I'm one of those doctors who needs to put labels on people in order to get paid. But it's possible to think differently. It will just take some practice until we all get it right — doctors included! Remember that we cannot skip Principle 1, *Be Present*, to arrive at this place. Dis-

PRINCIPLE 3: BE HEALTH | 103

traction will disempower us from making our own choices. The ego, judgments, and messaging of our current healthcare system endeavor to stop us from understanding what we must do for health practice, so we must first *Be Present* in silence if we're to find health.

Nor can we skip Principle 2, *Become Aware*. When we're aware, we gain a deeper understanding of the motivation behind the messages we're hearing. We begin to empower ourselves through knowledge and clarity. We begin to make our own choices, albeit perhaps difficult in this context. We are no longer victims of *health-fear* and begin to practice health instead.

In the next section, let's take a further look at how doctors love to label us with diseases, and how this diseased thought environment can restrict us from being health.

Disease Labels

Take a moment to answer this question: **Who are you?**

Are you Doug, Jack, Linda, Betty, or Cheri? Are you diabetic, hypertensive, or do you have Lyme disease? Or are you Frank the Diabetic, Jack the Stroke Victim, Linda with Lyme Disease, Betty the Brain Tumor, or Cheri the Colon Cancer? Do you sign your name on a credit card slip like that? Who exactly are you?

We are not these disease labels, just as we are not our thoughts, ideas, and beliefs. We are not even our names. Our names are labels, created for the purpose of easily communicating with each other. But we are much, much more than our labels. Our thoughts create an environment which we can more easily perceive, and therefore use, as a context from which to operate. They help us make sense of our world, our interactions, and each other. They serve as a reference point — but reference points can change. Perceptions can change. And so, when a doctor labels you with diabetes, hypertension, stroke, or cancer, must you automatically identify yourself with these labels?

"But they are real!" you may insist. "These are real diseases, and people need to pay attention to them." Doctors, in turn, may say that dismissing the significance of these devastating, epidemic diseases is tantamount to malpractice.

Is it?

104 | THE 7 PRINCIPLES OF HEALTH

These are nothing more than disease labels. They are no different than the guy in Walmart with the name tag that says "Hello, my name is John." What if a tall skinny guy and a short bald man were both called John? They have the same label, don't they? Shouldn't they be the same, then?

Just like our names, our diseases are not the same, regardless of what doctors may say. No two diseases are alike. They may be called by the same name in each individual, but they are not you, and you are not them. You are not Doug the Diabetic, Betty the Brain Tumor. You are you. And as you, only you should determine the next step you want to take.

Now, like many other conditions, diabetes does come with physical signs and symptoms. And ignoring those things can certainly lead to the worsening of your health and eventual death. So diabetes is the name of a type of health challenge. This challenge, however, is no different than a challenge you might face regarding a boss who's about to fire you or a late payment on your mortgage. It's just is a bit closer to home — your only home, so to speak. The thing to remember is that you can approach your health challenge objectively, just as you would a pending job loss or home foreclosure. You have choice about how you will react. Here we encounter that gap again, the point after defibrillation between the action and the stimulus when there is infinite choice. When the boss calls and says, "You're fired!" you may be understandably shocked, tearful, or angry. But do you go around telling people, "Hey, I'm Sharon the Unemployed" or "Just call me Rob the Late Mortgage Payment"?

More likely, after we've experienced an emotional reaction, we take a deep breath and say, "Right. Now how am I going to deal with this challenge?" You may argue that diabetes is not like a late mortgage payment or a job loss. It's a devastating, lifelong disease. That's true. But it's really the degree of fear behind the perception that makes it so devastating. If we are more fearful about the label of diabetes but less fearful about our job loss, we may say that diabetes is a death sentence but a job loss is not. Again, consider those who were diagnosed with cancer but survived. They didn't consider their diagnoses as death sentences. Those diagnoses might have been, though, by our current disease-focused model. They just weren't as stable as diabetes

PRINCIPLE 3: BE HEALTH | 105

with many options for treatment. Yet the survivors made the choice not to become the disease label called cancer.

It all comes down to our perceptions of our disease labels. Our perception is what we think; it's our thought environment. Our thoughts program our brains, which then trigger our belief systems, actions, and attitudes. These then manifest into our reality. They become real for us. So it can safely be said that we are what we think we are. If we believe right here, right now, that we are health, what are we? What will we become? What can we create, simply by thinking it is so?

Principle 3 tells us to *Be Health*. Period. We are and we will *Be Health* — right here and right now. It's just a matter of practicing saying those words until we believe them. And then our beliefs will dictate our actions toward optimal health in every instance.

●

Jerry sits behind me in class. He's about four foot one, give or take an inch, bent at the knees, waist, wrists, and spine, and he seems to be packed into the most amazing supersonic wheelchair I've ever seen. He asks me what I do for a living.

"Oh, I'm in healthcare," I toss off, casually. Our conversation circles back to him. "What's your diagnosis, Jerry?" I ask.

He smiles. To me, he's all face and square teeth, with tiny spastic fingers and a pair of Doc Martin feet that seems to stick out from his neck. A young nurse sits next to him. "I was born with spinal muscular atrophy.[26] But I've got a degree in communications, I was valedictorian of my class, I've been an international inspirational speaker, I've written several books, and I now work as a web content manager for a large tech firm in town."

"Oh." There's an awkward pause. "How did you ... please tell me your story."

"When I was born, they told my parents I wasn't going to be able to do much, that there was no cure for this disease. But I never believed it. I always believed I could do anything I wanted. I never saw myself as disabled."

"Really? What did your doctors say?"

---

[26]An inherited muscle-wasting disease

106 | THE 7 PRINCIPLES OF HEALTH

"You know, I was blessed with a really great doctor. He told me the diagnosis, but then he said, 'You know, Jerry. This is what you have, but this is not who you are. You don't have to be this disease. You can do anything you want, you know.'"

Ego and Judgment in Medicine

Not only are our own minds capable of criticizing just about everything we do, think, and feel, our egos can also lead us to make judgments in the context of healthcare. In particular, it's very disconcerting when doctors pass judgment. This is the line where objective science and subjective opinion diverge.

Why is this of concern? As supposed experts, doctors give advice. But if they first pass judgment or confront us with their massive egos, rather than using objectivity regarding our healthcare, we miss valuable opportunities for alternative ways to heal. Do doctors intend to do this? In most cases, they don't. But they, too, have programmed their thoughts to conform to The Current Health Paradigm. They too, have placed themselves inside very small boxes, surrounded by disease-focused thinking and practice. They attempted to prescribe health from within the confines of that box. We're beginning to see that this paradigm takes a very myopic or narrow-minded view of us as humans, doesn't it?

As much as doctors like to separate themselves from you, their patients, it turns out we are just like you, mainly because of the mere fact that we are also human beings! But sometimes a doctor's ego conveys the perception that he or she is separate from you. Whether your particular doctor is or isn't close-minded, the point is that you need to recognize their ego and judgment as such, particularly when it arrives in the guise of health advice. At those times, you must discern for yourself what you will do with that advice and make your own decisions. A doctor's ego and judgment about alternative healing modalities that are outside his or her experience or understanding could close many doors to your ability to find optimal health. Recognizing this fact and having the strength to stand up for your own decisions despite your doctor's opinions is a primary key to finding health.

PRINCIPLE 3: BE HEALTH | 107

Eckhart Tolle, author of *The Power of Now*, discusses the subject of ego at length.

The more you are identified with your thinking, your likes and dislikes, judgments and interpretations ... the stronger the emotional energy charge will be, whether you are aware of it or not. If you cannot feel your emotions, if you are cut off from them, you will eventually experience them on a purely physical level, as a physical problem or symptom.

It can be very difficult to identify where clinical evidence ends in medicine and opinion and judgment begin. Unfortunately, many doctors believe that their recommendations are always based on solid scientific evidence. Many believe their recommendations are the gold standard of medical practice and that anything else is condemned. They are often correct — but not always. When these recommendations become narrowly focused dogma that is shrouded in ego and opinion inside a disease-obsessed healthcare delivery system, you will become exactly what we all have become — full of disease. Doctors typically do not make any allowances for other methods of healing practice, and subsequently they cut their patients off from optimal health. Unconsciously, the very doctors who are supposed to help us heal may, in some instances, lead us into states of non-healing simply because of their own ego and judgment.

Consider acupuncture. This health practice, as you may know, originated as part of the ancient Chinese medical systems. Many people today actively seek out acupuncture as a way to help them heal, alongside conventional medical practice and applications. Many doctors even advise their patients to use acupuncture to help them heal, although technically, there is no scientific evidence to support this practice. Conventional medicine doesn't really understand how acupuncture works. We cannot explain the sequence of intricate events — how the superficial insertion of a fine needle into our skin can affect a particular protein or hormone, which in turn triggers a feedback response that sets off a series of events that eventually leads to the patient's healing. Nevertheless, we are now actively incorporating this ancient practice into "modern medicine." Many conventional practitioners now claim "medical acupuncture" as the new standard.

108 | THE 7 PRINCIPLES OF HEALTH

As a result, acupuncture is now almost considered mainstream medicine. But had you asked a doctor 10 years ago if he or she would recommend acupuncture as an option for their patients, you'd have received a very different answer. And today, some doctors still regard acupuncture with skepticism or ridicule. Recall my colleague's comment about our acupuncturist being a "voodoo" practitioner. What kind doctor makes a statement like that? Is it based on scientific evidence, or is it simply ill-founded judgment and opinion?

> *"If you think you can do a thing, or think you can't do a thing, you're right."*
>
> — **Henry Ford**

Let's consider a few other ideas. What about energy healing? What about intuitive guidance, quantum energy practitioners, astrologers who are mapping the brain to their practice, light therapists, past-life spiritualists, chakra healers, and clairvoyants? Are these practitioners to be written off by "mainstream medicine" because there is no scientific evidence to support their work? Should they therefore have no place in the healing art of medicine? Should a conventional medical doctor advise his or her patient who has found emotional benefit from these "unexplainable" techniques of healing to stop pursuing these treatments, even though they've caused no obvious physical or emotional damage to the person — and, in fact, have proven beneficial? If we project ourselves 10 or 20 years further into the future, will these therapies still seem ridiculous or fantastical, as acupuncture was perceived 10 years ago? Or will they be considered mainstream?

If we are to practice health, Principle 3, *Be Health*, tells us right from the start that we must not close our minds. We must not allow our egos — or the egos of our health providers — to dictate our path to healing. We must understand that the judgments and opinions of conventional medical doctors are founded in their own fears or insecurities. In the end, we must define for ourselves what will be our own unique path to health. And on the flip side, we physicians need to pay attention to what we're saying. We need to listen to our patients and truly hear the advice we are giving them, rather than just blindly move through our days, burning out from the weight of formulaic scripting inside a healthcare paradigm that's dying, along with our profession.

PRINCIPLE 3: BE HEALTH | 109

This is the only way we can hope to save our patients, ourselves, and our medical system.

Take a moment to identify your reaction to what you've just read. Are you angry or emotional about what I've said as a doctor or as a patient? Are you amused? Do you think I'm a quack or feel scornful or afraid of any conventional medical doctor who might recommend techniques you consider "having no scientific basis" and that you therefore believe should not be used? Are you familiar with the emotional, physical, financial, and spiritual benefits patients are finding through alternative treatments that they use in conjunction with allopathic medicine? Do you realize that many patients are already seeking this kind of care, but may simply not be telling their doctors for fear of judgment or ridicule?

Is such a reaction your own ego at play here? Is there another way you could see things? If we're all to find our way to health, both as doctors and as patients, we must begin to recognize how these kinds of prejudices and opinions in our healthcare system have kept us sick and removed from our ultimate purpose — to heal. Once we're able to navigate the maze of a medical system that seeks to close doors to health and healing, we can learn to stand up for all the alternatives that will help us find health. We will learn how to practice health and not medicine.

Letting Go

Let's face it. It's very, very difficult not to relive our past. Most of us have an active conversation going in our heads about actual events and fictitious episodes that may or may not have happened. Sometimes, as our minds continue to relive the past, our perception of things changes and we recall them as much better or much worse than they actually were. We may rewrite our personal history, remembering things people didn't actually say about events that happened and creating a revised version of reality. If we discuss a past event with someone else who was there, we may argue about our differing versions of the story. This is quite typical of human perception. Our "reality," as you can see, is very malleable. It can change inside our own heads, based on the day, time, place, or our mood. This, then, begs the question: is what we're recalling *actual* reality or is it just *our* reality?

110 | THE 7 PRINCIPLES OF HEALTH

What about the future? It hasn't happened yet, but in our minds, we plan things, think them through, fantasize about how events will play out, imagine what she's going to say, rehearse what we'll say in response. We project images of the future in our minds and live inside them. This triggers emotional responses in our bodies that may lead to real or imagined physical symptoms. We can become very sick, even needing to be admitted to the hospital, just by worrying about the future.

Our minds are very powerful. They can catapult us out of now. They take us to a past that's over and that often has become distorted into something that wasn't reality. They shove us into a future which never occurs exactly as we imagined. In sum, our minds prevent us from releasing past and future nonevents.

What does this have to do with healthcare? Much of our programming comes from the past. It's really quite scary how much weight we assign to our past. These messages come from traditions, culture, society, families, experiences, and our own internal attitudes. They often live with us for many, many years. We consciously or subconsciously build an entire repertoire of actions, thoughts, and attitudes around them.

Fear is a great example. Take someone like David's friend in the earlier story who lost both his parents. He now carries a tremendous amount of fear, which dictates his attitudes and belief systems regarding health and medicine. He feels that receiving a rubber stamp "You're healthy!" from a medical professional means he'll survive. But as we've learned, this tremendous fear and anxiety he's carrying around, although it's not showing up on the doctors' radar or list of diseases, actually means he's not living in health. He's unable to *Be Health*, as Principle 3 teaches us to do. He may for a short while feel relief that the doctor pronounced him healthy, but his chronic stress and anxiety over illness and death continually rear up, causing him to seek medical care time and time again to relieve the fear. We would probably agree, then, that David's friend isn't really healthy, is he?

If we are to find health, *Letting Go* has to be a part of our practice. As we've discussed before, most of us cannot just "let go" of so much material — years and years of programmed messages we receive at many different emotional and subconscious levels. How are we supposed to suddenly wake up one day and just release it all?

That is why the practice of *Letting Go* is exactly that, a practice. In order to practice this discipline, as we've stated before, we cannot skip steps. We cannot not skip the practice of being present through a technique like meditation, where our thoughts calm down and the prewritten messages stop. We cannot not skip the practice of becoming aware of what our medical system does to our messaging system and how it keeps us in a running commentary of fear, distraction, guilt, blame, sabotage, and victimization.

Once we are consistently able to practice Principles 1 and 2, we can proceed to our practice of Principle 3, *Be Health*. We do this by noticing when we are living in the past and releasing that thought — whether we're driving to work, talking with someone on our cell phone, or writing an email when these intrusive "past" thoughts invade our present. We do this by recognizing when we are fantasizing and living in a future of nonevents. We practice releasing every moment of every day. For the rest of our lives, we continue to practice. Don't get discouraged if it seems difficult to start! The more we practice, the better we get at recognizing these sabotaging thoughts or scripted messages, standing up to them, pushing them away, and returning to our present moment.

Yes, it does get easier with time, just like everything else to do with health.

YOUR INVITATION TO PRACTICE HEALTH

How can we help ourselves practice *Letting Go* in every instance?

I invite you to create something I call a Personal Health Mantra™. A mantra, according to the ancient yogis, is an instrument of thought that brings us back to the present moment, which is essentially our source of healing. When we create a mantra and recite it daily, we remember what we are, where we are, and who we are. We can program our brains with new thoughts and, subsequently, new actions that will serve us much better in health. Recall again that which is elevated in our minds has the power to manifest outwardly. This includes our abil-

112 | THE 7 PRINCIPLES OF HEALTH

ity to heal. A Personal Health Mantra can help us to let go and remind us of who we really are: a person and not the disease labels doctors love to give us.

Here are a few statements to consider when thinking about formulating your own Personal Health Mantra.

1. In this moment, I am: _____

2. I choose to: _____

3. I accept: _____

4. I know that: _____

As you complete these statements, you may want to consider them in the context of your health. If the exercise still seems vague or difficult for you, don't despair! You are welcome to visit health-conscious.org and view a copy of my own Personal Health Mantra as an example.

Accepting

As mentioned earlier, finding our way to optimal health by using *The 7 Principles of Health* requires that we practice *The 5 Disciplines of Health Practice*. We've already seen how fear plays a great role in our lives and how we must find health by dismantling the fear. We've also discussed ego and judgment in medicine and how they can close doors to healing providers who practice outside mainstream medicine. Now let's take a look at another discipline we all need to learn: acceptance.

●

Doctors often forget people's names when they talk to each other about their patients. It's not an insult; it's just part of the training. We remember our patients by their disease labels.

"Remember the leg in four? Well, he died last night from a pulmonary embolism."[27]

"Hey Jackie, after you're done with your pâté, can you take a blood sample from the liver in three?"

---

[27] A blood clot that has traveled to the lungs

PRINCIPLE 3: BE HEALTH | 113

"Josh, I've got a migraine from that headcase on med-surg![28] *Why didn't you tell me to turf her to psych?"*[29]

Leonard was a "lung" I met while doing an emergency room (ER) shift in a small town in Canada. He rolled into the ER in a wheelchair, panting like a puppy.

"Shawn!" I exclaimed nervously to the male nurse. "What's this guy's O2 sat?!" Shawn didn't seem worried. He pushed the patient into a curtained room, helping him out of the chair and into the bed. He then began hooking him up to monitors and machines.

I stared at the angry, blue-grey man in front of me. His face was carved in frown lines. Shawn strapped an oxygen mask over his mouth and nose, and the blue faded into what must have been his normal color — leathery yellow.

"Seventy-six," Shawn said calmly. "You've got an oxygen sat[30] of 76 this time, don't you Leonard?" Shawn asked, raising his voice.

Leonard's scowl deepened. "GODDAMN YOU!" he erupted in a muffled voice from behind the mask. "JUST DO YOUR ... GODDAMN ... JOB. STOP PREACHING ... AND GET ME ... OUTTA HERE!" He couldn't speak more than two words without gasping for air. He turned his eyes on me. They were piercing black and didn't seem to match his sallow skin. "WHO ... THE HELL ... ARE YOU?!"

"That's our new doctor," Shawn replied. "She's from Alberta."

"ALBERTA, EH? ... COULD'A ... FOOLED ... ME!" Leonard said, sizing me up. "IMMIGRANTS! ... TOO MANY ... IN THIS ... COUNTRY!"

"That's enough," Shawn said sternly, looking up from the IV catheter[31] he was about to insert into Leonard's arm. "Or I'll make it really hurt. Trust me."

"JUST GET ME ... MY DAMN ... DRUGS!" Leonard bellowed.

"What does he usually get?" I asked Shawn. "125 of Solu-Medrol® and a nebulizer?"[32]

---

[28]Medical-surgical floor in a hospital

[29]Psychiatric floor in a hospital

[30]Measure of a patient's oxygen level that is used to determine if they are low on oxygen

[31]Intravenous catheter

[32]A machine that delivers aerosolized medication through the lungs as a patient breathes

"Sometimes they give him three or four. He's had it all — albuterol, aminophylline, Atrovent®, steroids[33] — you name it. What he needs is a new set of lungs. Don't you Leonard?" Shawn threw the needle into the sharps container. "I'll be back with your drugs. Be nice to our doc."

By this time, Leonard was breathing a little easier. His eyes seemed to darken into two ebony dots. His lips spread over seriously tobacco-stained teeth. I was about to lean over and examine him when he shouted again.

"I KNEW IT!" he said with a scornful tone. "DON'T KNOW WHAT YOU'RE DOING, EH? WET BEHIND THE EARS?"

I felt my face flush. "Leonard? How much do you smoke? Two, three packs a day?" I tried to soften my voice and sound caring, but truthfully, I felt as though he deserved to be this sick, especially since he was so nasty.

"THIRTY-FIVE YEARS!" he declared adamantly. "DON'T BOTHER TO ...TELL ME ... TO QUIT! GODDAMN IT! THEY ALL DO!" He shot a threatening glance at me and then turned his head to the wall.

Shawn returned with a nebulizer and syringe filled with milky white steroid. He pulled down the IV port and began to push the liquid into Leonard's veins. "Got a set of grocery bags in there, don't you Leonard?" He tapped Leonard's chest. It sounded hollow. I could see the spaces between his ribs suck in with every breath. "How many visits here this month? Three? Four?"

I shot a surprised look at Shawn.

"Has he been on a vent?[34] We'll have to transfer him down to the city."

"He won't go," said Shawn, shaking his head. "Right, Leonard? You won't listen to us, will you? Gotta do your own thing, eh?"

"I AIN'T ... STAYING IN THIS SHITHOLE!" He jerked is arm from Shawn's fingers. "OUCH! THAT HURT! ... CAN'T YOU PEOPLE DO ANYTHING RIGHT?!"

Shawn raised his eyebrows and grabbed Leonard's arm to stabilize it. He finished pushing the meds and cleaned up. He adjusted the drip rate on the IV and then turned to me. "If you need me, Doc, I'll be in triage."

---

[33]Medications that are commonly used to help someone with lung disease

[34]Ventilator machine that helps patients to breath artificially

PRINCIPLE 3: BE HEALTH | 115

"Thanks, Shawn." He disappeared, leaving me alone behind the curtain with Leonard.

"THE HELL IF I'M GOING IN AN AMBULANCE!" Leonard declared, eyeing me suspiciously. He hesitated for a moment. "WHY ARE YOU HERE?"

The way he said "you" made me cringe. "I'm replacing Dr. Jones for a couple of weeks. What about you? Why are you here?" I couldn't help dragging out the word "you."

"AIN'T IT OBVIOUS?!" Leonard growled. "WHAT KIND'A DOCTOR ARE YOU ... ANYWAY? LOOK, JUST HURRY UP ... AND GET ME ... THE HELL OUTTA HERE!" He began to swat at the mask on his face.

"I think we'll have to admit you for a few days," I said. "You need to be stabilized."

"HELL IF I'M STAYIN'!" Leonard pronounced fiercely. "I FEEL BETTER! LET ME OUT!"

The curtain pulled back and Shawn poked his friendly face inside. "Where do you think you're going, tough guy?" he asked.

"GET ME A GODDAMN CAB!"

"Settle down," Shawn said, adjusting the sheets and pulling up the bed rails. "We'll let you go in a moment, as soon as these medications are done."

That was Leonard, the Lung.

I told him to quit smoking or he would die soon. I told him if he smoked at home with an oxygen tank, he would blow up. I told him not to be so rude to people.

"I DON'T GIVE A SHIT ABOUT ANYONE!" he bellowed. "LET ME GO HOME TO MY GODDAMN CAT!"

He left the emergency room, against medical advice. He came back a few days later and we repeated the same song and dance. He left again, against medical advice. He came back again. It seemed he had memorized my schedule. His medical records showed he was admitted to the emergency room only on my shifts.

Every time he came in, he was breathless, angry, and blue. He would leave angry and yellow. But slowly, over the course of a month, his color began to change to a pasty ash, despite all the treatment we gave him. He lost weight, and his arms and legs turned into leather skin on bone.

116 | THE 7 PRINCIPLES OF HEALTH

One day he came in, doubled over in the wheelchair. He wore a dirty T-shirt and green cotton sweats that hung in loose folds from his body. We did our song; we did our dance. We gave him drugs and set up machines that would help him breathe. But Leonard's lungs didn't want to breathe for him anymore.

Later that morning, lying on the gurney,[35] the mask over his face, Leonard slowly opened his eyes. He turned his face toward me.

I shivered as a cold chill went up my spine. Gone was the piercing black I remembered from just a few weeks ago. His cheeks and eye sockets had sunk into his skull. But it was his eyes. His eyes had changed. I felt like I was staring into the eyes of a living ghost.

As he lay there in front of me, cracked lips, wrinkled skin, he began to speak in a hoarse whisper. "Thank ... you, Doc," he croaked, lifting a weak finger and touching my forearm. "You're ... a good person." He closed his eyes. "Thank ... you."

●

In the end, we will all die. We must accept that, as there's no way around it. We can choose to fight as hard as we can. We can stress ourselves out about it. We can worry about it every day. We can pay corporations to tell us they can do something to prevent it or sucker us into believing they can protect us from it while they siphon our money. But however hard we may try to avoid the fact of our own mortality, our end is death.

Once we accept this fact, we can breathe into Principle 1: *Being Present*. We can *Become Aware* of who's lying to us, as shown in Principle 2. We can *Be Health*, as Principle 3 teaches us, right here and right now. And in those moments, we will find that we have the amazing power to choose a different way to live; without worrying about a future that may or may not happen, without reliving the past again and again, and without damaging our physical bodies through the fear, distraction, and disempowerment that surrounds us in today's medical system.

The question, then, remains: *What will you choose?*

---

[35]Hospital bed commonly used in the emergency room

YOUR INVITATION TO PRACTICE HEALTH

I invite you now to try a brief exercise to help incorporate some of the discussion points I've raised in the previous sections. Doctors use medical charts, each of which contains something called a *problem list*. This list itemizes the diseases with which you have been diagnosed. Here is a sample problem list taken from a real patient.

1. Overweight (BMI — 27)

2. Type 2 Diabetes Mellitus

3. Hypertension (high blood pressure)

4. Hypercholesterolemia (high cholesterol)

5. Hypothyroidism (low thyroid)

6. Vitamin D Deficiency (low vitamin D)

7. Premature Ovarian Failure (early menopause)

8. Anxiety and Stress Disorder

9. Chronic Low Back Pain

10. Myopia (nearsightedness)

Take a moment to answer one question: ***Do you think this patient is sick or healthy?***

Gary Null says in his book, *Power Aging by Gary Null*, that in the absence of disease or discussion about disease, when we pursue wellness in its many forms, disease corrects itself. Keep your answer to the above question in mind for a moment as we move on to discuss one last thing.

The Final Choice is Yours

Our human bodies are innately designed to heal. Each of us contains a healing source within us. The ancient Chinese practitioners called

118 | THE 7 PRINCIPLES OF HEALTH

this healing force *qi* (pronounced "chee"). The ancient Indians called this force *prana*. What they believed about illness or disease is that these channels of life force become blocked, resulting in a state of *dis*-ease. Healing practitioners would reopen these channels and allow the body to tap into its own source of healing, and the life force would flow once again.

Somewhere along the way, we forgot about *qi*. We distracted ourselves with medicine after medicine, test after test, and fix after fix. We suppressed our energy flow by grasping outside ourselves for health. We began to rely on others to show us the way, and in the process, we distracted our own bodies from their ability to find their intrinsic healing energy source.

There's almost always a chasm between what we are and what we can be. There's a difference between what our society and healthcare system have programmed us to be and what we can create ourselves to be. When we begin our journey to find ease and health, we begin in health, right here and right now.

In conclusion to this section on Principle 3, *Be Health*, please recall the medical problem list taken from the patient's chart earlier in the chapter. I would like to share with you that these are my problems, taken from my own medical chart. I believe that despite these health challenges, I am healthy. I live in health, every day. While I know that I will die one day, perhaps sooner than many without the disease labels given to me by the medical profession and the fears instilled in me by our healthcare system, I choose to live in happiness, joy and health, right here and right now.

Remember, no matter what your diagnosis is, you always have choice because you are life. Learn how to *Be Health* in every moment of it!

CHAPTER SIX

Principle 4
Reawaken Curiosity

"You'll miss the best things if you keep your eyes shut."
— **Dr. Seuss** *(1904-1991)*
American author, cartoonist, and artist

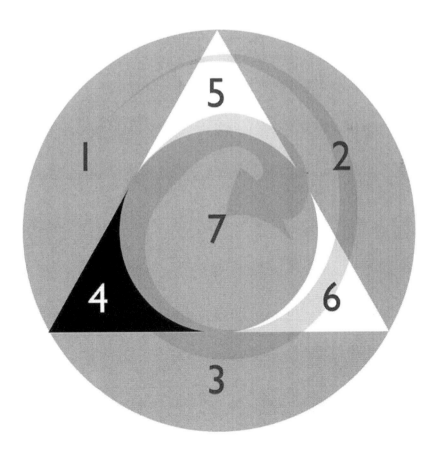

120 | THE 7 PRINCIPLES OF HEALTH

We learn many things as we grow older. But when it comes to caring for our health, curiosity is something many of us have lost.

Have you ever watched a 2-year-old run into a room full of toys? What does he or she do? At first, our toddler may be shy or scared and hang about his mother's legs. But soon he feels safe and begins to explore. The bright colors and interesting shapes attract him. He wants to play with other children. He begins to laugh, run, pick things up, and turn them over in his hands. He awakens his natural sense of curiosity and learns from his environment, without prejudice or pre-conception. While his brain is processing information, he's changing. He's developing his sensory, motor, and cognitive systems through his curiosity and interaction with his world.

We were once that same toddler, exploring things with innate curiosity. What happened to us after we grew up? Somehow, caught in the crazy pace of modern society, working too hard, and displacing our true priorities for material gain, we began to churn the treadmill of life and we became dull. We became content to sit in front of the T.V. and stare.

When it came to our personal health, we seemed to retreat even further. We waited for the government to serve Medicare and state-run healthcare programs that left us no incentive to maintain our health. We waited for employers to offer us private health insurance. We learned to believe that if we ate what we wanted and didn't ex-ercise, someone would still take care of us at the end of the day. We bought into messaging that told us that drugs or procedures could fix us if anything went wrong. And when something did go wrong and we were harmed, we sought compensation from the help of all-too-eager lawyers. We became more curious about the features on our new iPads and iPhones than we were about our own health.

As we've been establishing, the networks created for us by health insurance companies, so-called "health networks," are not really health oriented. They are actually disease networks, wearing health disguises. Both doctors and other providers who are accepted into these net-works are told how to practice (i.e., DIAGNOSE DISEASE) or they won't get paid. They are paid to deliver disease care, so that's what they do.

The health system basically stifled our sense of curiosity about our health. It told us what we needed to prevent, treat, fix, and cure

PRINCIPLE 4: REAWAKEN CURIOSITY | 121

disease. Health seldom even entered our conversations. Our thoughts, actions, and belief systems were focused away from health and toward trying to prevent disease or, if we were unlucky, trying to fix it. We kept searching for cures instead of learning about optimal wellness. We became diseased because we were not curious enough to learn about health practices. We believed the way to health could be found by fixing disease, even if there wasn't a fix.

●

Margaret stares at me.

"I don't think you need a prescription for antibiotics," I tell her. "You've had these symptoms for only one day, and all of them are consistent with the common cold. That's typically caused by viruses. Antibiotics don't work against viral infections."

"So what am I supposed to do?" she says in a frustrated tone of voice. "I know I'm going to get worse. It happens to me every time. The five-day pill works the best. It fixes me the next day."

"But taking a drug comes with potential side effects," I reply. "In fact, it might prolong your illness. Using too many antibiotics has caused resistance, and we're running out of medications to treat people."

"Well I'm different. I want you to prescribe, what is it? Zithromax®?"

"Would you like me to show you the *Physician's Desk Reference* on that drug? It has a list of all the potential things that can go wrong, even if you've taken it before. If you don't need a drug, which I'm telling you is unnecessary, why would you want to take it anyway?"

"Because that's what they've always given me! And it works just fine for me."

"But I'm telling you that you don't need it. In fact, it may be harmful. And you still want me to prescribe this pill?"

"Yes I do. I paid to see you and I want my prescription."

"So let me get this straight. You want me to prescribe a drug for you ... for absolutely no reason?"

She stares at me with a blank face. "Yes."

Fear and Curiosity

What has our dulled sense of curiosity done to us? This is really a chicken-and-egg question. Have we stopped being curious because of the medical system and its doctors who have been conditioned to say they'll take care of us? Or have we stopped being curious about disease because we've focused so much on the cure that it scares us to know more about things which have potential to kill us? Regardless of which occurred first, our dulled sense of curiosity about health has kept us sick on many different levels. And it all seems to arise from a deep sense of fear which, as we've discussed, is the foundation of our healthcare system and its way of operating. As a result, we've become more content to sit back and let someone else take care of us.

Because we learned to focus on disease and became afraid of disease, we stopped being curious. We spent most of our time on the fear of disease. Since we were not guided toward health as a crucial component of healthcare, and as a result lost interest in it, we also stopped learning how to practice health in a significant way. We breathed a sigh of relief, thinking "the system" would take care of us, and we would therefore remain healthy. We believed a healthcare system like ours could manage our health because it promised to fix our disease.

On the flip side, doctors were kept in fear, too. How might a doctor learn to be afraid? One way was learning that we would not be paid for practicing health instead of disease inside a system that focuses so much on disease care. Doctors practice defensive medicine first because of their fear about getting sued. They're afraid of violating mandates or being accused of fraudulent practices by a bureaucratic system that justifies its existence by first finding fault with physician practice. Doctors are afraid of being kept out of disease-focused health insurance networks and are afraid that patients will not come through the door if they teach health instead of disease. And they are afraid of being accused of not knowing enough about the practice of health by patients who are seeking healthcare options, like Patricia with her breast cancer diagnosis.

But the reality is that doctors don't know how to practice health. They've been trained in the practice of disease. Their extensive 10+ year education isn't about how to eat properly, exercise, rehabilitate

PRINCIPLE 4: REAWAKEN CURIOSITY | 123

the body, mediate, or heal emotionally and spiritually like other practitioners who begin first with this paradigm. Conventional doctors are trained in understanding, diagnosing, and then working backward to find cures, fixes and screening tests for disease.

In addition, America is overrun by specialists who spend an extra three to five years after medical school in their chosen field, examining the minute details of a particular organ or system. They learn how to diagnose, treat, fix, and cure very rare diseases. They don't learn about the common illnesses that plague the general population or how to recommend total health as a starting point for optimal health management. They learn how to break the human body into its mechanical parts rather than viewing it as a series of integrated, whole, energetic systems. This is the difference between Newtonian physics and Einstein's physics theory. Doctors consider physiology down to its molecular, cellular, and protein levels. They attempt to map genomes or manipulate an endless array of diseases through gene splicing, promising that we can find health this way. Yet they don't understand the intricate multidimensionality of who and what we are as human beings.

So doctors become fearful of honest health questions because they have the potential to reveal that the doctors themselves, as disease-trained specialists, are inadequately trained to teach or practice health. Preprogrammed messages delivered via institutions, by virtue of education and training, ego and judgment, have been used to disguise this fear so that you, the patient, won't realize that most doctors simply aren't trained to know anything about integrated health. How can they when all they know how to do is break apart the human body into mechanical parts?

And instead of collaborating fully with quality alternative and complementary practitioners, learning and opening their minds out of curiosity so that they can offer you options as a patient, they have in the past polarized or separated medical practice. They have fragmented medicine into conventional and alternative practices, or Eastern and Western medical systems. They unknowingly bought into the programmed messages of a broken, separated health system, dictated by outside parties interested only in profit. They believed this was the right thing to do in the name of health. They didn't know how to shift their own perspectives enough to stand up against these parties who

124 | THE 7 PRINCIPLES OF HEALTH

were toxifying the relationship between them and their beloved patients.

Stephen Covey calls this scarcity mentality. Scarcity mentality is based in fear. In medicine, we call it turf wars. Conventional doctors pit themselves against alternative practitioners, and vice versa. Each uses derogatory comments when discussing the other. Collaboration is shunned and you, as the patient, are caught in the middle. "I'm not going to send you my diabetics!" says a family doctor to the chiropractor who's attempting to network with her. "They're my bread and butter." Is this her way of saying that she needs to keep her patients sick in order to make money inside a system that has trained her to keep them sick?

> *"Children are remarkable for their intelligence and ardor, for their curiosity, their intolerance of shams, the clarity and ruthlessness of their vision."*
>
> — **Aldous Huxley**

I recently had an argument with a general surgeon about the business of medicine. He questioned our clinic's model of collaborating fully with massage therapists, chiropractors, acupuncturists, and naturopaths.

"You're just shooting yourself in the foot," he said to me.

"Does that mean we, as doctors, don't want our patients to get healthy?" I asked him.

With shrinking dollars, healthcare expenditures that are skyrocketing well into the trillions, and a medical system that's long broken, we all need to think differently. We each need to learn about health, both doctor and patient. We need to take matters into our own hands, reawaken our curiosity, and do our homework. We need to talk with health professionals of all types and learn from them, not just the ones we've been conditioned or programmed to believe are health providers. We all need to change the paradigms from which we operate.

Principle 4, *Reawaken Curiosity*, teaches us that, in the end, we are the only drivers of our own health, not the external stakeholders we have, until now, allowed to make decisions for us. We are the decision makers. And to do a good job, we all must first be curious about health. That means remembering what it's like to be a kid again, running into a room full of toys.

Requirements

A good place to begin to reawaken our innate sense of curiosity might be in understanding a few minimal requirements. These are things we must have before we can truly change. *The 7 Requirements for Health Practice* are fundamental attitudes and processes which each of us must understand in order to find health. If one of them is missing, we will never heal. We simply won't be able to. And no one else can help us or make us heal unless we first come to the table with these basic requirements. Recall *The 7 Requirements for Health Practice* outlined in the first chapter.

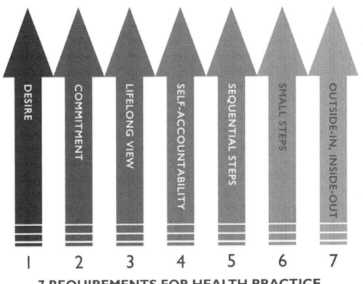

7 REQUIREMENTS FOR HEALTH PRACTICE

In the next section, we're going to discuss each requirement as it is listed above. Then we'll examine the difference between curiosity and distraction, and why it's important to understand the difference. Lastly, we will explore how distraction can lead to desperation and, paradoxically, the inability to find health, especially when we're suddenly faced with a terminal illness.

Requirement 1: Desire

Desire is the attitude we possess when we want something. We can't tell someone, "Please desire this for me." They might really want us to have that shiny new car or to live a little longer because they love us dearly, but they simply cannot desire our wishes for us, no matter how much we may want something to happen.

Our medical system has somehow taught doctors that they are responsible for their patients' health in almost every instance. Notice I didn't say disease. The healthcare system will never imply that a doctor is responsible for someone's genetics, which can contribute to their disease manifestation. But it does hold doctors accountable for their patients' health, or lack thereof, despite the fact that the doctor has to operate inside a disease-driven medical construct.

When health insurance companies realized they were paying a lot of money for expensive technology and procedures for the people they insured, they began to look for ways to control costs. One way to control costs was to examine the risk factors for a person's health problem. For example, if uncontrolled high cholesterol and obesity caused a patient to require an expensive cardiac bypass, the health insurance company would examine the doctor's practice to see whether he or she had fixed their patient's cholesterol value or helped them lose weight. Doctors who had patient populations with excessively high cholesterol and obesity rates wouldn't get paid if their patients' cholesterol wasn't lowered or if their patients didn't lose weight. In other words, the doctor would be punished for their patients' health conditions by the health insurance companies who paid them.

Recently, the same thing has begun happening with America's Medicare program which refuses to pay hospitals if patients are re-admitted with ongoing illness, but who won't and can't find adequate healthcare outside the hospital, because Medicare refuses to pay those doctors, too! In these situations, doctors are also not paid for teaching or counseling patients on health. Their only resort, then, was to threaten their patients that they would get sicker and die if they didn't fix their own diseases. Doctors had to pass down to their patients the punitive measures the health insurance companies and government programs were inflicting on them.

PRINCIPLE 4: REAWAKEN CURIOSITY | 127

Regardless of bureaucracy or economic incentives, however, who is the only person who can change you? Even if your doctor begged you every day to lose weight, could you do this if you really didn't want to? Could he stop you from running to McDonald's that night because you were too busy to have time to eat properly?

> *"In order to succceed, your desire for success should be greater than your fear of failure."*
>
> **— Bill Cosby**

Now let's take this a little further. In hearing your doctor make ominous comments in his or her office — beginning with predicting disease, and followed by the threat of getting sick and dying from that disease — would you feel guilty about stepping onto the scale? Would you be tempted to blame your genetics, your spouse, your kids, your stress, your job, or anything and everything else you could think of? Might you consider buying McDonald's that very night because you felt so badly about yourself that you just didn't care, or you thought it would be too difficult to change? These questions are not meant as judgments. These are normal emotional reactions. Paradoxically, guilt, blame, and sabotage are expected emotional responses to punitive measures inflicted by doctors (and all the other stakeholders we've mentioned in this book) under a healthcare system that uses this technique to badger you into finding health — and the system perpetuates their conduct. In the end, it's really a vicious, paradoxical circle that spins you in every instance, towards getting sicker.

It's not the doctor's fault. It's not the patient's fault. It's not even the health insurance company's fault. It's a hidden irony, embedded deep within the context of a profit-driven healthcare system. Someone has to pay. Someone has to save money. Someone has to show results. The health insurance company targeted the doctor as responsible for showing results, whether their patients wanted to change or not. But the doctor had absolutely no control over whether their patients desired the mandated change.

As we can see, desire is a fundamental requirement to finding health. And it's got to be *your* desire. *You* have to want to change. No one can make you change, not even a doctor who has put the fear of disease and death into your mind. You have to want change for yourself.

Requirement 2: Commitment

It's not enough, however, to desire to change, even if it's born from fear. There must be commitment, as well, and that commitment must come from you. We all may have the desire to lose weight or change our health in some way, but until we commit to ourselves — not to our wives, husbands, children, doctors, or dogs — we'll never change for life. Desire and commitment are best friends when it comes to our health. They go hand in hand, everywhere. One without the other will likely result in failure.

It's sometimes difficult to be committed, let alone being committed to change in today's highly distracted world. With national divorce rates topping 60 percent, we can't even commit to each other as husbands and wives. It seems that nothing is sacred anymore.

That's why, in order to commit to health, Principle 1, *Be Present*, becomes so important and is worth another mention. When we are present in the now, when we take time to be silent, we commit. Silence is golden, they say. More than that, it must become sacred to us. Commitment is the simple act of stopping the disempowering distraction, coming back to the present moment, even if it's just for one minute a day. So without doing anything as complicated as creating a bunch of spreadsheets, graphs, goals, and calculations, we can commit through the simple act of turning off the white noise of our world through one minute of silence a day. It's that simple, but that difficult.

Requirement 3: Lifelong View

Health practice manifests health. And remaining healthy is a lifelong endeavor. That's why health is for life. It becomes the very definition of life, doesn't it?

When we want to shift our point of view toward health (desire) and we carry out the initial step to doing so (commitment), we also need to understand that we're in it for the long-term. Unfortunately, in modern society and medicine, the word "long-term" creates a great deal of anxiety. It's really the opposite of what we've been conditioned to do and what we've done in healthcare — attempt to speed things up.

PRINCIPLE 4: REAWAKEN CURIOSITY | 129

Take a look at the events of 2008. The entire stock-market bubble was an example of a short-term business outlook. Now go back in time. The dot-com era was another example of our short-term mindset. Go back again. The Medicare bankruptcy threat we face today is another example of a short-term construct. In the sixties, no one expected our population to grow and age as it has. We're now living the results of such short-term vision. All we have to do is look at just about any event in our history to understand that our practices and habits often stem from short-term viewpoints. Wars, environmental damage, Wall Street crashes, unethical corporate practices, food shortages, population explosions, illness, famine, genetic manipulation, and the rise and fall of nations all stem from short-term perspectives.

> *"Tell me and I forget.*
> *Teach me and I remember.*
> *Involve me and I learn."*
>
> — Benjamin Franklin

Perhaps it's because we're only human and feel that we should do as much as possible within our short life spans. With this perspective, however, we end up accomplishing much less than we could have. Those with a broad understanding and long-range plan are the most successful. It's the same with our personal health. When we commit for the long haul, we practice health in every moment of every day. We practice for life. We live for health. And then, we don't end up with the escalating numbers of diseases that plague us today: clogged arteries, arising from greed and a quick-fix mentality; degenerative joint diseases, which stem from our obese bodies; and stress-related illnesses, which are killing us emotionally and physically. All of these began with a short-term, quick-fix mentality.

Principle 2, *Become Aware*, helps us understand that health is not the result of a quick fix and never will be. We must understand that today's medical system will continue to perpetuate this viewpoint, because short-term profit supersedes long-term health when the motive for health management is profit driven. It's only when we, as individual patients and doctors, stand up for change by choosing a long-term perspective that we will begin to truly reform our health care system from disease obsession to optimal health practices.

Requirement 4: Self-Accountability

Being self-accountable means we report back to ourselves. We become honest with ourselves. We hold ourselves to a higher standard. We seek only the best when it comes to our personal health. We don't do it in response to our doctors' threats of disease or death; we don't do it in response to health insurance costs; and we don't do it because the government mandates us to get healthy. We do it because it matters to us.

Self-accountability is a natural consequence of desiring a positive path for our health, and then committing to that practice. No one else can make us change, as we've discussed before. When we want to do things for ourselves and when we commit to doing them, we are, by definition, self-accountable.

Take a moment to read these messages:

"My doctor said I have to _____."

"If I don't get this test or procedure done, my doctor says _____ will happen."

These are words of fear and victimization. These are the words we use when we allow outside forces to determine our health. We may decide to change because we feel threatened or afraid, but the change will never last because we did not do it for ourselves.

So let's examine the very basic example of Mindy. At five feet five and 250 pounds, she's a woman at risk for many things, including heart disease and diabetes. If she were to say, "*My doctor told me to diet and exercise,*" how much would you bet that she'd stick to a program and actually accomplish her long-term goal? The diet and exercise industries make billions on yo-yo dieters and weekend warriors.

Now, what if Mindy were to use *The 7 Principles of Health*, as I've outlined them in this book? She might begin by telling her doctor, "Okay, I've got a few health challenges, but I'm not going to see them as disease (Principle 2, *Become Aware*). Right now, I feel fine (Principle 1, *Be Present* and Principle 3, *Be Health*). So I'm going to identify a few things I can do to practice health (Principle 4, *Reawaken Curiosity*)."

So Mindy signs up for a new women-only pole dancing class. She's embarrassed at first, but after a few weeks, she starts laughing with the other ladies and realizes they were also initially embarrassed. Before

PRINCIPLE 4: REAWAKEN CURIOSITY | 131

she knows it, Mindy is already feeling better in her skin. She hasn't lost weight yet, but she's confident and happy. She feels empowered. So she tosses aside the judgments of her family and ex-boyfriend, who say pole-dancing is for strippers; she ignores the judgment of her doctor, who says pole-dancing isn't really exercise — and guess what? After a month, she's lost 10 pounds! Not only that, she feels so good that she listens to her common sense telling her that McDonald's isn't going to work for her anymore. It makes her feel bad, and she doesn't want to feel that way anymore. She starts making different choices with her nourishment. No, she doesn't start a "diet" like her doctor told her to do. She just makes different food choices.

> *"Change before you need to."*
>
> — **Jack Welch**

In two months, Mindy's down 20 pounds! She begins to dress differently. She acts differently. And she's not bouncing up and down on the scales with her weight anymore. Do you think she would have accomplished any of that if she'd kept telling herself, "My doctor says I have to diet and exercise"?

When we are accountable to ourselves, we succeed because we do it for ourselves. We have choice. There is no other way to health.

Requirement 5: Sequential Steps

Life these days can be overwhelming. The next requirement for finding optimal health is following each step in sequence, and learning how to implement it. When we follow *The 7 Principles* in sequence, each builds on the prior and makes our journey to health easier.

For example, we cannot understand that we have become highly distracted by medical messaging today if we haven't mastered Principle 1, *Be Present*. If there is no time for silence in our day, if we don't stop the white noise, we cannot rise high enough to see the forest from the trees in our quest to find a new perspective. If we aren't aware of how the health system has actually been designed to keep us sick, as I've outlined in Principle 2, *Become Aware*, we will continue to be deluded into equating a static checkup for the absence of disease with optimal health. These can be difficult concepts to digest, espe-

132 | THE 7 PRINCIPLES OF HEALTH

cially in light of such a tightly woven ideology as we have been led to believe inside today's healthcare system.

It may take some time for you to truly be able to step away from the distraction, to empower yourself, and to operate from a different viewpoint in order to continue your journey to health. The system, even if you intend to proceed toward health, is designed to pull you back into its disease-focused mindset by its very nature. That's why another requirement for health change is to follow the steps in order.

This doesn't mean we can't repeat some of the steps, or go back to practice them again and again. In fact, it will be necessary to retrace our steps. Each time we do, we will understand something a little different about ourselves and our bodies. We will see something different about what's happening around us. We will begin to realize that there is a new way to act and think. We go back and, like staring out the window of an airplane that's rising through the clouds, we see things as they actually appear, just from a higher altitude.

Requirement 6: Small Steps

Our society loves to go from 0 to 60 miles an hour in 3.2 seconds flat. Things have sped up and seem to be getting even faster by the day. We talk fast, we eat fast, we text fast, and we live fast. We get frustrated because we can't go faster. And then we die fast.

People reading this book might think, "I don't have to follow *all* these steps, do I? I'm going to skip Principle 1, *Be Present*. I'm already present. Besides, I'm so busy, I just don't have time to stop and meditate. That's for those yoga-granola hippies. Why isn't Natasha just telling me what I have to do to get healthy?"

My reply would be: *Go ahead and try skipping to the end. Finish the book and set it aside. Read it, but don't actually take any action. See how just reading it works for you. Notice what happens in your life. Take a few notes. Have you changed in any significant way? Are you beginning to think differently about things you believed were true in health, but may somehow seem incorrect right now? Do you feel like you've achieved your health goals? Did you do it in order to make your doctor happy or to prevent disease?*

Make no mistake — the prevention of disease is important. But contrary to the popular belief that it will lead us to health, it doesn't.

PRINCIPLE 4: REAWAKEN CURIOSITY | 133

This process still begins from the same paradigm that's been keeping us sick. We're attempting to start from the fear of disease in an effort to make ourselves healthy. Until we change that mindset via the small-step progression of *The 7 Principles of Health*, we will never stick with health as a long-term view.

As I've outlined in *The 7 Principles* and *The 5 Disciplines of Health Practice*, the steps to health are like a baby learning to

> *"Be the change you wish to see in the world."*
> — **attributed to Mahatma Gandhi**

run. Babies are born without the ability to walk or sprint out of the womb, no matter what an admiring parent might say. It's just the way the human body is made. And so, just like babies, we must all continue to take baby steps to find health for life. There is no other way, especially given what our traditional healthcare messages and programs have trained us to believe. If you want to find lasting health, taking baby steps will be a fundamental component of reaching that goal.

Requirement 7: Outside-in, Inside-out

It is important to understand that we've been working from the outside in. Typically, it's best to change from the inside-out. We must first change ourselves in order to change the world around us. So why am I advocating change initially from the outside-in?

We must change from the outside-in because we operate from inside the healthcare box that we've constructed as The Current Health Paradigm. When it comes to how we live, it seems that greed, profit, and power become so entwined in the discussion that our fear of death jumps to the forefront of our minds, clouding our subsequent decisions. Unable to act, we simply react. Unable to see things clearly, we buy into the threats and punishments. We cede to authority, unable to question it and do whatever the stakeholders tell us to do. We act like the victims we've allowed ourselves to become.

Changing from being a victim to one who is empowered, like Patricia, Allison, Pastor John and many other patients have done, requires an unbelievable amount of courage. We begin our journey to change and find health with Principle 1, *Be Present* and Principle 2, *Become*

134 | THE 7 PRINCIPLES OF HEALTH

Aware. We begin with the courage to sit down and listen first. But what are we listening to? We are listening to ourselves, our common sense, and our own truths about what is right and what is wrong for us. We are listening to new information that tells us we don't have to buy into the reality we think we see. We have the choice to see something very different, including whatever we wish to see for our personal health and future.

According to the Indian spiritual and philosophical writer, Jiddu Krishnamurti:

> Society does not want individuals who are alert, keen and revolutionary, because such individuals will not fit into the established social pattern and they may break it up. That is why society seeks to hold your mind in its pattern, and why your so-called education encourages you to imitate, to follow, to conform.

It will take a tremendous amount of courage to move away from a basis of fear and operate from a new paradigm, especially when it comes to the future of our health and healthcare system. Much is at stake — not only your own personal health, but the entire deconstruction of the The Current Health Paradigm and the channels we've long been trained to follow in order to find health. I believe we cannot hide from this change any longer. It's a matter of our health, our lives, and the world we wish to leave behind for our children. If we are unable to find the courage to change and heal ourselves first, we will never be able to change our world. So, in the context of health today, we must begin from the outside-in.

From there, change will naturally flow from the inside-out.

●

Tracy suffers from extreme stress and anxiety these days. She's beginning to feel the physical effects of her out-of-control life. She tells me she has fluttering in her chest and wakes up in a cold sweat most nights, gasping for air. She can't fall asleep because her mind races. "I burst into tears at the drop of a pin," she says, reaching for a tissue in my exam room.

"There are pills that can help your symptoms," I tell her. "I'd be happy to prescribe them for you. But have you ever considered a dif-

PRINCIPLE 4: REAWAKEN CURIOSITY | 135

ferent form of treatment that might help, one that doesn't require you to take a pill?"

"No. What do you mean?" she asks, drying her eyes.

"I've been talking with Dr. Bowen. She's a Doctor of Oriental Medicine who was trained in China, and I've learned a lot about the many different conditions that acupuncture can treat. Anxiety and stress, believe it or not, are among them. I know, it may sound odd. I didn't know that myself until I spoke with her. Instead of using pills, which can

> "If we don't change, we don't grow. If we don't grow, we aren't really living."
>
> — Gail Sheehy

make you sleepy and have addictive potential, would you consider trying acupuncture? I've been amazed at some of the conditions Dr. Bowen has been able to treat." I wince, "Even I didn't believe it would work, but it does."

Tracy's anguished face stares back at me. I can see in her emerald eyes that she's almost lost hope. "I'll try anything," she says. "Anything." She buries her face in her hands.

A few weeks later, I pass Tracy in the hall, and I almost don't recognize her.

"Oh, Doctor!" she exclaims excitedly. "I want to thank you so much for helping me. You know, I didn't fill the Xanax® prescription you gave me. I hope you're not offended. But I'm so glad I didn't. I felt so awful, but I just didn't want to take a pill. So I went to see Dr. Bowen, like you suggested, and oh my, she's helped me so much! Things haven't changed in my life, but I'm sleeping better and I can cope so much better! I'm able to sort a few things out with a clear head now. Thank you for referring me."

Tracy then wrote the following testimony of her experience:

I was taking Prozac daily for anxiety and had run out. I went to a local clinic to see the doctor and renew my prescription. I was told they would not see me because I had an outstanding bill. (I explained that I was a cash patient and that I paid per visit ... how could this be?? No one had any answers). I drove [to your clinic] desperate and in a full-blown panic attack. ... At that point, I was willing to try ANYTHING! At your suggestion, I returned to the clinic and had a consult and first

136 | THE 7 PRINCIPLES OF HEALTH

treatment with Dr. Bowen. I had not considered acupuncture before, but I was glad I did this ... because the panic attacks stopped almost immediately after the treatment began. I have not had a panic attack since the beginning of my acupuncture treatment. The bottle of 30 Xanax® pills is still full. ...You saved my life!

Some people, doctors and non-doctors alike, may roll their eyes and say that this experience didn't really "save" her life. But I ask you to reconsider. What is life, after all? Is it the ability to merely exist from disease state to disease state, from pill to pill, from fix to cure to disease to attempted fix to cure — again and again in a vicious cycle from which we can never escape? Or could life be much, much more than what we've been programmed to believe, not necessarily a long time, but a top-quality time here on Earth?

The way we perceive things determines our reality. To find health, we'll need to change our perceptions, open our minds, and reawaken our curiosity to learn new things every day and in every instance, just like we did when we were kids.

YOUR INVITATION TO PRACTICE HEALTH

Let's take a moment to see if we might step away from our egos and judgments to learn how to open the doors to our personal healing practice.

The following exercise will require you to "listen" to your immediate reactions, those you feel in your body (e.g., a surge of adrenalin in your gut in response to what you read) and those you can "hear" yourself saying when you're really paying attention. It might be a good idea to repeat the sentences aloud to yourself immediately after you've had a reaction (sort of like counting to 10 before replying to that email that's irked you). Sometimes, when we slow things down and really listen, we can hear where preprogrammed messages have played a role in the medical system and our subsequent inability to find health.

PRINCIPLE 4: REAWAKEN CURIOSITY | 137

1. Think of a health practice with which you are familiar. If you can't think of anything, you might use one of these as an example: *bioenergetic healing* or *quantumpathic* or *energy matrix healing*. Don't think too hard. Just write down a response as quickly as you can, even if you find yourself saying, "That's not really health related."

_____

_____

2. Next, write down your immediate reactions to that word. Try to name three things, perhaps describing a feeling you notice yourself having.

_____

_____

3. Repeat these words aloud. Really listen to them. Try and identify whether they are programmed messages, and if so, where they might be coming from (e.g., your own thoughts, based on your belief systems or attitudes (internal locus or reference point), or from something you might have read or heard someone else say in the past (external locus or reference point).

4. Next, do what America does best: Google the word and see what happens.

5. Read at least three different resources about this word. For example, you can use Wikipedia, an Internet article, or someone's website. Just read the information. Don't worry whether it's scientific or not, for now. Try and be as objective as you can about what you are reading.

6. After reading these three sources of information without judgment, do you think this healing practice might be a safe, effective way to help someone heal (emotionally, physically, spiritually, mentally, or even financially)?

138 | THE 7 PRINCIPLES OF HEALTH

Curiosity and Distraction

What is the difference between curiosity and distraction? Let's take a look at Catherine in the example below.

Catherine is an uncontrolled diabetic who has amassed years of bad eating habits. She's come into an acute care center, for lack of a better place to find health.

"Is caffeine bad for me, Doc?" Catherine asks. She's obese, with high blood sugar, well over 300 today. "I think I might have to stop drinking coffee."

"What are your usual eating habits?" I ask.

"Oh, I know I ate too many sugary things over Christmas. But it was Christmas, after all. And we had a lot of company. And I guess there was Thanksgiving before that. The kids came home from out East. But what about soda pop? Do you think if I stop drinking Coke, that'll fix my diabetes?"

"Coke has a lot of sugar, yes." I reply.

"But I love Coke. Do you think if I choose the caffeine-free, sugar-free version, it will help me lose weight?" She looks imploringly at her husband.

"You really like to drink Coke," he nods and then looks at me. "What do you know about Avandia®?[36] Do you think she should be on that drug, Doc?"

Catherine chimes in before I can answer. "We wanted to go out together for breakfast today. What do you think if I have an omelet? What kind of omelet should I have, Doctor? Oh, but I love sausage and bacon. I can't skip those today," Catherine says.

"No. You can't skip the sausage today," agrees her husband. "We haven't been out to eat together in quite a while. Maybe you can skip the sausage next time, but not today." He smiles lovingly at her and then turns to me. "What about metformin?[37] She was told to take metformin by another doctor. But we didn't fill the prescription because I've heard it can be bad for you. What do you think? Is it good or bad?"

"I can't stand broccoli," says Catherine brusquely. "But they say asparagus has lots of antioxidants. Maybe I could add a little asparagus

---

[36]Avandia® is a prescription drug used to treat type 2 diabetes.

[37]Metformin is another prescription drug used to treat type 2 diabetes.

PRINCIPLE 4: REAWAKEN CURIOSITY | 139

to my omelet. Dr. Oz says cabbage is good — what's it called — bok? Bok choy, right? He says that's really good for you. I read in the news that if you eat a lot of asparagus, it will help prevent cancer." She turns to her husband. "Oh, Jim, we're going to the restaurant with the buttermilk pancakes. Mmmmm, remember those, honey? Weren't they the best we've ever tasted?"

Catherine truly wants to change. She's curious about health. She watches Dr. Oz and reads the news. But something crucial is still missing in her approach to health.

●

Our sense of curiosity often leads us to surf the Internet. We're curious about So-and-So's recent love scandal, the disaster in Japan, what the political candidates are saying, and how peanut butter may directly or indirectly correlate with heart disease. We filter these pieces of information into sound bite form and then move onto the next topic. We sift through the latest studies and listen to all the media hype about finding health through the fear of disease. But no one, so far, has been able to truly synthesize our approach to health amidst this incredibly distracting environment.

Doctors can't help us synthesize information about health, no matter what the experts may say. In fact, doctors perpetuate fear through disease-focused training inside a disease-focused paradigm, unintentionally, as we've discussed. They teach us to find health by checking for disease, and then teach us only to prevent disease, rather than informing us about how to seek optimal health or making the time and acquiring the expertise to help us with our behaviors and habits. Health insurance companies find no value in encouraging you to find a behavioral or nutrition coach who might be central to your health. Instead, they tell you to visit the doctor and screen for disease via "regular checkups."

Curiosity, as it applies in Principle 4, must have a sense of purpose. That sense of purpose is embedded in a much larger picture of medicine than the one we're currently able to see. In Catherine's example, she and her husband are distracted by asparagus, Coke, Dr. Oz, omelets, and metformin. They are trying to get her weight under control and find health, but they are ignoring the bigger picture, which

140 | THE 7 PRINCIPLES OF HEALTH

includes her attitudes and long-term behaviors. She uses social events as an excuse for her eating pattern, and then seeks to find health by correcting one specific detail. She cannot see that even if she quits drinking Coke but continues to eat the way she has been and then engages in blame, she will sabotage her long-term efforts and will never find health, perpetuating her role as a victim.

It's not Catherine's fault. It's just that she has been programmed to seek health by distracting herself with pills and the details she hears in the news. She may amass an endless list of things that could help correct her diabetes. She'll try one new thing after the other, or follow the advice from the latest study or from Dr. Oz she's just heard about on T.V. But it doesn't matter what the latest study or Dr. Oz tells her. The only way for her to find lasting health is with purpose. And her overall, big-picture purpose should be to correct the deeply engrained habits that are killing her slowly.

Unfortunately, our current medical system is unable to help her. Through distraction, it will paradoxically keep her sick. By paying disease-focused providers — specialists who know disease inside and out but haven't been trained in health behavior or in a health-oriented paradigm — she will remain ill. They will first recommend diet and exercise, but leave her to figure out how to do it on her own. Next, they will prescribe pills to distract her from the underlying behavioral support she needs but is not getting. When she tries to engage someone to support her, she'll find that those costs are not covered by her health insurance, despite the thousands of dollars she is paying to "stay healthy."

Principle 4, *Reawaken Curiosity*, teaches us to focus our curiosity so that it leads us to see a bigger picture. To find health, our curiosity needs to bring us to practices of health first, not down the road, a subsequent step to chasing disease prevention. This is the big picture. Medicine's advocacy for preventing disease first is noble, and although correct from one aspect, it is the wrong place from which to find true health.

PRINCIPLE 4: REAWAKEN CURIOSITY | 141

Curiosity and Desperation

"Can you call Frank?" my personal trainer asks me. "He's been diagnosed with terminal prostate cancer. His wife trains with me. She was asking for options. It sounds like they're desperate."

"What did his doctor say?" I ask.

"That there's nothing more to do," she replies. "But he's so desperate, he'll try anything at this point. I didn't know what to tell them, so I thought I'd ask you."

●

This is the end point of a fix-it, cure-it medical system, the point at which none of us wants to arrive. This is the point we reach when we've failed to face our fears, let-go of our past programming and the messages that bombard us daily, take baby-steps to practice health in every moment, and accept our lives, our diseases, and our death. This is where Frank, although he's still living, will spend every breathing moment he has left, trying desperately to push away his fear of death. And this is the point that will lead him to die long before he breathes his last.

Our curiosity can lead to distraction if we are unable to see the big picture first. Worse, our curiosity and distraction can result in desperation when another variable, like a terminal disease diagnosis, is introduced into the equation. Modern medicine seems to enable us to slip into desperation very quickly. Because many of us have relinquished our power into the hands of The Current Health Paradigm and its practice of disease labeling, we have become victims of it. And when we find there are no more answers, we no longer have the tools within ourselves to find health, and our fears take over. We cling to the disease-focused system for hope until, suddenly, the doctor's exam room door slams closed. Our questions are now met with irritation, as if we've become nothing more than a bother. Like Pastor John, we're told to choose our coffin and go home to die.

As long as we continue to distract ourselves, we will never become empowered to make our own choices. And as long as we remain free of terminal conditions, we won't worry too much and won't seek to change. We might read this section on curiosity, glancing over

142 | THE 7 PRINCIPLES OF HEALTH

the concept of distraction and desperation with amusement, thinking, "I'm glad that doesn't apply to me." I completely disagree. It applies to every single one of us, healthy or not. Because inside a medical system that's based in fear, disempowerment, and distraction, a system that's driving both the healthy and the diseased toward more sickness in all five components of health (mental, physical, emotional, spiritual, and financial), it will only be a matter of time before we all become desperate. And by that time, as in Frank's case, it may be too late.

The Paradigm Tables Revisited

Let's see where we are in relationship to The Current Health Paradigm and The New Health Paradigm from earlier in our reading. Take a moment to read these words. Has their meaning changed for you?

Again, circle the words that seem to resonate with you as you read them aloud. Now that you've come this far, you may have a very different understanding of health. You may be able to see that some of our current healthcare perspectives will no longer serve you well in your journey to health. The old institutions will no longer be able to help you. It's a bit scary, but you must be willing to acknowledge the fact that you are on your own when it comes to finding health.

The Current Health Paradigm	The New Health Paradigm
Quick Fix	Long-term
Fragmented	Whole
Individualistic	Collective
Cure	Heal
Disease-oriented	Health
Mechanical	Energetic System
Polarized	Balanced
Victimization	Empowered
Paternalistic	Guide or Teacher
Mandate	Collaborative
Blame	Accountable
Judgment	Nonjudgmental
Myopic	Clear Vision
Unconscious	Conscious

PRINCIPLE 4: REAWAKEN CURIOSITY | 143

Our medical system has been broken for a long time, but we've been deluding ourselves into thinking that our elected officials or promises from for-profit stakeholders can help us heal. They can't. Not when our illness is a fundamental requirement for their existence. Not when disease is necessary for them to make a profit. Remaining as victims inside this current healthcare system keeps us from finding true health in our bodies, minds, spirits, and personal finances.

Principle 4, *Reawaken Curiosity*, has brought us one step closer to this understanding. But what are we supposed to do when we're buried under the weight of so many complex ideas? How are we supposed to find health in our society when we are constantly told by our health insurance companies to stay within our contracted provider networks?

In the next section, we'll learn about Principle 5, *Channel Creativity*. You may ask what being creative has to do with health, medicine, and disease. Actually, it has everything to do with our health! Specifically, we're going to talk about the creation of our own health networks. Instead of going to visit doctors who have agreed to contract with health insurance companies and must practice under the current disease-focused system, we will learn to make another choice. In every moment, we have choice. Recall the diagram from Chapter 3: *Stimulus, Gap, Action*. Between the stimulus and the action, there is a gap, which is our ability to choose.

So we can choose to visit health practitioners who are in alignment with The New Health Paradigm. We can choose to create networks of only those providers who will show us the way to health, correct our diseases through health, and support our love of life, regardless of our health challenges. There's no reason we must continue to accept the disease networks of for-profit health insurance companies any longer. We can and should make a different choice for our health.

Robert Kiyosaki, in his book *Rich Dad, Poor Dad*, tells us that we should each create our own personal network of financial and legal advisors in order to find wealth. Most of us wouldn't keep a bookkeeper around if we knew they had been embezzling our money and sickening our personal finances for years, would we? So why do we keep visiting doctors who continue to operate within a drug-prescrib-

144 | THE 7 PRINCIPLES OF HEALTH

ing paradigm, thereby keeping us sick? Why do we hang on to providers who don't offer us personal choices in our pursuit of health, who simply dictate treatments to satisfy their own egos?

We all have this power, even if not immediately apparent. We needn't worry about how much it's going to cost, either. There is a way to create a unique, personalized health network that costs almost nothing. This concept is called a *Health-Centric Model*™ and refers to a healthcare model which begins from a paradigm of health, not disease, as we shall discover in the next chapter. And once we truly shift our paradigm toward health, we will fully understand that paying trillions of dollars into disease networks that falsely promise health no longer serves our needs.

YOUR INVITATION TO PRACTICE HEALTH

I invite you to open your eyes, as Dr. Seuss has advised us, and *reawaken your curiosity!* Log onto health-conscious.org and check out the amazing health practitioners I have met on my journey. These practitioners are *Health Conscious Movement* approved. In other words, they operate from a health-oriented perspective that seeks to view you as an integrated being. They offer unique ways of finding balance between physical, emotional, mental, financial, and spiritual health.

Contact any one of them to schedule a visit, and learn how they can help you heal. Use this as part of your research as you journey toward health. Keep your mind and heart open. You're welcome to interview as many different providers as you'd like! Do your homework! Reawaken your curiosity! Become a toddler once again and learn, learn, learn how to find your way to true health!

CHAPTER SEVEN

Principle 5
Channel Creativity

"What we think determines what happens to us, so if we want to change our lives, we need to stretch our minds."

— **Dr. Wayne Dyer** *(b 1940)*
American psychologist, author, and motivational speaker

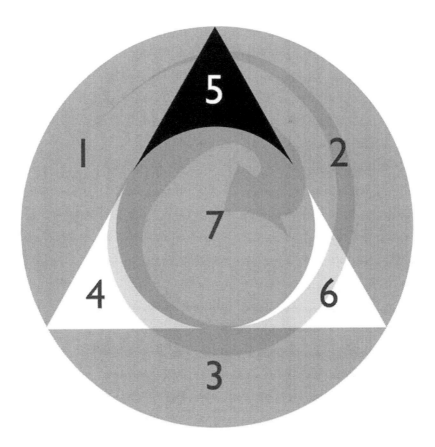

146 | THE 7 PRINCIPLES OF HEALTH

We like to think artists are creative, that they have a talent or gift for sharing their designs with the world. We describe writers who paint word pictures or dancers who show us different forms of expression via body movements as creative. Neuroscientists have found that creativity originates mostly from the right side of our brains. This area houses our spatial, visual, and intuitive abilities.

For some reason, however, we don't tend to describe health as a creative endeavor. Doctors will agree that there's an art to medicine, but our modern healthcare delivery system will not allow the art of medicine to be monetized. We operate deep inside the left, scientific half of our brains, which requires explanations, proofs, calculations, and technical formats in order to make things logical so that we can believe them.

YOUR INVITATION TO PRACTICE HEALTH

Let's take this moment to try a quick exercise. Take a blank sheet of paper or open a new Word document on your computer.

1. Think of all the health providers with professional degrees you've seen or will see. For example, write down the names of your primary care doctor, cardiologist, dermatologist, or pulmonologist. If you have a chiropractor or naturopath, write their names down, too.

2. Next, write down the names of any therapists you may have seen or will see. For example: physiotherapist, massage therapist, acupuncturist, or reflexologist.

3. Take a moment to look at the list you have created. Beside each name, jot down whether the person is a conventional (Western or modern medicine) or alternative provider (Eastern or holistic medicine). It doesn't matter if you're right or wrong; just put down your first impressions.

PRINCIPLE 5: CHANNEL CREATIVITY | 147

4. What do you think about your list of disease or health providers? Is there a balance between those you've labeled as conventional and those you've labeled as alternative? Do you have mostly conventional practitioners on your list? Do you have mostly alternative practitioners?

5. Take a moment to circle the most important person on your list, the one you would say is most likely to help you achieve optimal health.

6. At the end of the list you just created, add a few more lines. Would you add your personal trainer, nutritionist, herbal medicine practitioner, spiritual counselor, or pastor as part of this health network? Why or why not?

●

Lyn sits on the lime green chair beside the exam table in our office. She's in her late 40s, but her face is deeply creased with frown lines. She looks worried, stressed, and anxious. Her eyes are rimmed in red and she nearly bursts into tears when I say hello. I ask her what's wrong.

"I'm a personal trainer," Lyn says. "And I love what I do. I lead a very healthy life, eat really well, and exercise, obviously. My problems started about a year ago — I don't know why. I started to get achy all over: my back and thighs, mostly my shoulders and hips. I couldn't figure it out. I ignored it for a while but then I started having a lot of trouble getting out of bed in the morning. I'd have to take an ibuprofen just to get my day started. So I decided to see the doctor."

"What did he or she do?"

"He ran a bunch of tests and couldn't figure out what was wrong, so he sent me to a rheumatologist. I've seen that guy about six times so far." She slumps in the chair and looks down at her feet.

"What's he done? Did he give you a diagnosis?"

"No!" she exclaims in a frustrated tone. "Every time I see him, he just keeps ordering more and more tests. And when I tell him I'm in pain, he gives me a prescription. He's given me some hydrocodone[38], but I hate it. I can't function on it. I can't teach."

---

[38]Hydrocodone is a narcotic prescription medication.

148 | **THE 7 PRINCIPLES OF HEALTH**

"So why did you come to an acute care clinic?" I ask gently. "How do you think I can help you?"

"I don't know," she says dejectedly. "I had to quit my job because I couldn't teach anymore. Then I had to apply for coverage under my state-run health plan. They tell you which doctors you can see, and this rheumatologist is the only one on their plan. I'm not earning any money, and I don't know what to do. But I don't want to take those pain pills."

"What did your specialist say when you asked what's wrong? How does he plan to help you?"

"He doesn't say anything," she says, her voice cracking. "He just keeps mumbling and writing prescriptions. And then he rushes out of the room. I don't want any more prescriptions! I don't want any more tests! I want to see if I can treat things naturally, but they won't cover those kinds of doctors." She stops for a moment and snorts. "You know, every time I see him, he looks so stressed, like he's depressed. I want to tell him he should think about changing jobs. And he's really too young to be that burned out." She looks up at me. "Can you help me?"

My eyes slide to the closed door.

"I'm sorry," she says. "I didn't mean to bother you. I just don't know what to do. But I'm in pain every day. I tried to teach an elderly class the other day. I thought I might be able to ease back into work, maybe try it part-time. But I couldn't even do that. I don't want to get hooked on drugs. But I can't afford any other insurance. I don't have any money. And now I don't have a job."

●

Does it matter what Lyn's diagnosis is, especially if she seems to be getting worse despite six or more visits to a specialist who hasn't come up with an answer to help her heal? At this point, does her disease label matter, or could a different viewpoint from which to operate be far more beneficial? What do you think a doctor like me would advise someone who has no job and is not earning enough money for private health insurance, has a state-run insurance plan that won't allow her to seek help from alternative practitioners, and who is getting worse by the day, so much so that she's headed toward a dependency on

PRINCIPLE 5: CHANNEL CREATIVITY | 149

narcotics just to relieve her very real pain? Is Lyn's case hopeless or is there another way for her to heal?

There are innate forces inside each of us that have the potential to help us heal, no matter what the diagnosis may be. Modern medical practice has used countless prescriptions to distract us from tapping into that innate source, causing our bodies to work hard to detoxify those drugs instead of focusing on enabling ourselves to heal.

How does someone like Lyn even begin to navigate a medical system that is casting her deeper and deeper into a sinkhole that seems to be leading her straight toward disability, poverty, and addiction — even though she's trying desperately to find a different answer? If we

> "Creativity is just connecting things. When you ask creative people how they did something, they feel a little guilty because they didn't really do it. They just saw something. It seemed obvious to them after a while. That's because they were able to connect experiences they've had and synthesize new things."
>
> — Steve Jobs

seek to heal ourselves, we must become like the great artist Michelangelo, carving into our personal slab of marble in order to free our innate abilities to heal. This is the outside-in process mentioned earlier. But how do we accomplish such a feat?

Principle 5 shows us how to *Channel Creativity*. Instead of relying on the network of so-called "health" providers (disease-focused providers) dished out by health plans, we're going to actively seek those who can lead us to health by beginning from a different paradigm than the one modern medicine wants to keep us focused upon. In order to do this, we need to begin with practitioners and therapists who operate from a different perspective than that of conventional doctors. Conventional doctors operate from a position of "preventing" or "diagnosing" disease, and then attempting to fix it. In Lyn's case, her rheumatologist continues to search for disease, doing the same thing again and again, yet expecting a different result. Such behavior has been called the definition of insanity.

Complementary or alternative doctors begin from a different perspective: the human body is an integrated system of energy, while

150 | THE 7 PRINCIPLES OF HEALTH

disease is a manifestation of blocked energy flow, or *dis*-ease. They ask themselves, "What is the best way to unblock energy flow to release the life force within you in order to heal?"

Without jumping into the well-entrenched mindset of modern medicine and asking, "What's the fix, then?!" let's review Lyn's problem in the context of the five *Principles of Health* we have discussed so far.

Principle 1: Be Present

How much would it cost for Lyn to find one minute a day — right here, right now — to stop her current programmed messaging system she has been taught to believe in healthcare? The words she hears from her health insurance plan tell her she must continue to see doctors and specialists to manage her disease. But she doesn't have a diagnosis, and their management plans aren't working! So what is she supposed to do? If she called the insurance company and asked them, I'm sure they would tell her to ask her doctor what to do. And her doctors would keep prescribing different medications and ordering more tests. She might continue like this for years, getting worse every day. These messages would continue to spin in her mind, and she would continue to believe that following her doctors' advice was the only way to find health. But is it?

What if Lyn were to stop listening to these messages for one minute a day? What if she were to just breathe, stop thinking, and feel her body? What if she were to relax her mind and her body during these sessions? Do you think her high levels of cortisol, a very harmful hormone that's pumped by our adrenal glands during times of stress, would lower as she relaxed her mind and body? And could lower levels of this cortisol, which leads to chronic inflammation and is likely the basis of Lyn's muscle and joint pain, be helpful in alleviating some of her pain — even a tiny bit?

Principle 2: Become Aware

Of what must Lyn become aware, as it relates to her case inside the current health system? She's already aware of it. She just doesn't know how to say it aloud.

PRINCIPLE 5: CHANNEL CREATIVITY | 151

Lyn is very aware that the conventional medicine treadmill she's running on is getting her nowhere. She's not finding any answers by continuing to follow this type of advice. She's also aware that her doctors are burned out. They're so burned out that she's recommending they change professions. What is the likelihood that these doctors who are so dispassionate about their own lives and careers can actually care about Lyn?

> *"I saw the angel inside the marble and I carved until I set him free."*
>
> — **Michelangelo**

Principle 2, ***Become Aware***, teaches us to call things like they are. Lyn's not getting anywhere by continuing to search for disease; it's not helping her find health. She needs to stop and try a different way of thinking. She needs to do something different for herself. And she needs to have the confidence to stand up for herself and acknowledge what is happening, recognizing that she will likely find no further answers via her current efforts if she hasn't already found them after more than a year with a top medical specialist. Her answers don't lie in medical practice. She will find them only in her own personal health practice.

So far, Principles 1 and 2 have not cost a dime! Shall we continue to see how Lyn can help herself heal?

Principle 3: Be Health

As Lyn begins to turn down the volume of noise from the media, health insurance rules and policies, and doctors' narrowly focused, disease-oriented mentality, she learns to refocus her thoughts toward health. As she learns to practice silence, she introduces health mantras into her process which contain affirmations that she is health right now, in this moment. She is complete. Nothing is wrong with her. She doesn't need to keep repeating that she is sick and must prevent disease. She realizes that taking more and more pills for pain and other conditions without a plan for overall health is not preventing disease.

Lyn doesn't need to reinforce old negative scripts as part of her new thought environment for health. She simply has a few challenges that happen to be related to her health. One of those challenges is

152 | THE 7 PRINCIPLES OF HEALTH

pain, not a rheumatologic condition or a muscle condition or whatever other disease label a conventional doctor may want to give her. For the time being, her actual diagnosis is immaterial. First, she must deal with her pain in ways other than what conventional medicine has taught her.

Many famous people, like Dr. Wayne Dyer, Dr. Deepak Chopra, Eckhart Tolle, and Carolyn Myss, understand we are not pain and pain is not us. Pain is simply our perception. Our ability to cope with pain is malleable. If we internalize pain and identify with it, it becomes a significant part of us, and we may then experience it even more severely. But if we are able to separate ourselves from pain, to step away from it and mentally displace it, we can experience a less intense feeling. We can even reach a state where we feel entirely free of pain.

You might believe that Lyn has pain, that she's getting worse, and that she should do something more about it than sitting around meditating. You might think I'm being irresponsible as a physician to recommend that she stop and incorporate silence as part of her life when she's clearly suffering. Am I?

Is Lyn's situation critical right now? Has she tried just about everything known in conventional medicine, without finding any answers? Have people undergone surgical procedures without experiencing any pain, using only hypnosis or acupuncture? Is what I am recommending in Principle 3, *Be Health*, so fantastical that it shouldn't be tried, especially since there are no side effects?

Creating a daily space for silence in our lives doesn't generally cause bodily injury. It isn't a toxic drug with the potential for addictive or sedative side effects, or even the potential for death. If this technique can alleviate a significant proportion of Lyn's pain, and if she begins to feel better and require fewer drugs, couldn't we say that this practice is helpful to her health? And couldn't this practice be something that also has the potential to help the rest of us to heal? Do we need to wait until doctors or the FDA tell us there is "scientific evidence" that meditation is harmful or beneficial, victims of the paternalistic attitude we discussed earlier in this book, or should we proceed to do exactly what we all know is right for us to find true health?

Lyn's positively affirming thoughts and her practice of being still have led her to a place of calm relaxation and have decreased her pain levels. Although she still hasn't been able to return to work, she is finding that her mind is no longer spinning with worried, negative, or stressful thoughts about how she's going to find a cure. And her body is beginning to respond to health.

Principle 4: Reawaken Curiosity

Now that Lyn is a little more grounded and less stressed, she's become curious about finding other ways to heal. But she thinks she must spend money she doesn't have to book an appointment with a naturopath. Does she really need to do this?

What if Lyn were to attend one of the many free seminars that her local holistic practitioner hosts for the community? What if, after the seminar, she talked with the practitioner and he or she suggested using something natural, say a homeopathic remedy or vitamin supplement, or even foods that might reduce the inflammation in her body? What if she spent $5 on Amazon for a used book of natural remedies and learned how to treat her condition based on its recommendations?

Even though Lyn doesn't have a specific diagnosis, she knows she has inflammation in her muscles and joints. She knows it's probably some sort of rheumatologic condition. Should she wait another year or two for her doctor to figure things out, if he ever does, before she tries something different? What if the disease label turns out to be "idiopathic," which is a doctor's way of saying, "We don't know what's going on and we don't know how to treat it?" Or do you think that Lyn should begin to learn a few things about how to approach her pain by taking a new tactic? She may learn that changing her diet even further reduces the inflammation that seems to be causing the pain or find a few natural supplements or techniques like acupuncture that can help her. Or should she keep repeating lab test after lab test and taking drug after drug, only to achieve the same non-results again and again?

What if Lyn met an intuitive healer who worked with his clients' blocked energy fields? What if that energy practitioner had an upcoming group session for a nominal fee? Say Lyn finds such a practitioner and decides to attend that session. The intuitive healer finds that Lyn is still carrying around programmed messages from her childhood that

154 | THE 7 PRINCIPLES OF HEALTH

she hasn't yet released. It turns out that some of her deep-seated emotions are affecting her ability to heal and manifesting in her body as inflammation and muscle weakness. She's been suppressing these toxic energies all this time, never really dealing with them. Is this a crazy concept to believe, in terms of healthcare?

Lyn decides to work with the intuitive healer. Her pain decreases as she learns how to release the past. After a few sessions of energetic cleansing, she feels much better. She's healing her body by healing her mind. Should we, as doctors, claim that this is the work of a quack and do everything we can to stop our patients from seeking this kind of help because the scientific proof is absent; the government has told us not to do this; the health insurance companies won't pay for it; or the pharmaceutical companies tell us their pill works much better than this inexpensive natural option?

Insanity inside our healthcare system reveals itself at many different levels.

Principle 5: Channel Creativity

Lyn meets a holistic practitioner at a free seminar who suggests one or two things she might take to help her pain. Lyn finds this tremendously helpful. She also puts aside a small amount of money to attend group sessions with an acupuncturist and finds these to be very helpful, as well. She works a couple of times with an intuitive guide to help her release some baggage from the past that she's been carrying around with her all these years. She practices being present every day and tries to stop living in the past or the future. She also manages to teach three or four classes a week and resumes her position as a personal trainer at the college part-time. She's in less pain than before.

At the college, she meets a personal trainer who teaches plant-based nutrition, based on Dr. John McDougall's work. Because she works at the college, Lyn can attend this class for free. She modifies her diet, becoming vegetarian. She has found more help for her "medical" condition in these last few months, outside the conventional system, than she's found in 18 months of visits to "regular" doctors. While she still checks in with her rheumatologist once in a while, she now decides for herself which bits of advice will work for her and which

PRINCIPLE 5: CHANNEL CREATIVITY | 155

won't. She refuses to accept a "one-pill-fits-all" solution to her personal health issues.

What do these practitioners represent to Lyn: a holistic medicine doctor, a nutritionist, an acupuncturist, a medical intuitive, her rheumatologist, and her primary care physician? They make up her network of health providers and practitioners. Without investing a lot of money and by operating outside her state-run health insurance plan, which was inadvertently keeping her sick, she's

> *"A pessimist is one who makes difficulties of his opportunities, and an optimist is one who makes opportunities of his difficulties."*
>
> **— Harry Truman**

created her own network of health guides. She's stopped focusing on conventional medicine as having all the answers, and is instead learning to practice health despite her disease. She still follows some of the advice from her conventional medical doctors, but their advice is no longer the only solution Lyn has available to her. Nor are they exclusively responsible for her health.

Lyn has taken baby steps toward shifting her health paradigm. She's no longer operating from fear. She's operating from a very different perspective than the one she had when she first came to see me in the exam room. She now sees an opportunity for health, whereas before she only saw disease. Like Tracy in our previous example, Lyn has been shown a different way to see things, which has led to healing, choice, health, and empowerment, as well as a dramatic change in the quality of her life.

We have been blinded inside conventional medicine by our own egos, judgments, and opinions, as well as those of the system surrounding us. We have closed doors to healing and our minds to common sense. It will be up to individuals like Lyn to find their own way to health by channeling creativity through unique health networks like the one she has created for herself.

●

I now invite you to return to the list you created for yourself at the beginning of this chapter. What do you think of your network? Are there other health providers you might consider adding to your network,

156 | THE 7 PRINCIPLES OF HEALTH

now that you've read Lyn's story? Are there providers in your network who do not serve you well in health? Are you afraid that if you don't see them as you've been instructed, you will get sicker? Or have you actually become sicker by seeing them and regularly following their advice?

●

Jeff is a friend of mine. He's six foot two, muscular, and truly the poster boy for health. He's kindhearted and friendly, and when we chat, we always talk at length about our passion for health.

But Jeff is sick, very sick. He's got stage three Lyme disease.

"I started to feel like something was wrong when I was in college back East," he says. "I was on the football team and I started feeling pain. At first I just thought it was because I was playing hard. You expect to hurt a bit when you play ball," he grins. "But after a while, I started hurting more. I felt really tired all the time, more than I should. So what did I do? I trained harder. I didn't listen to my body and told myself I just wasn't working hard enough. But it was weird. I still got worse. So I finally went to a doctor."

"What happened?"

He rolls his eyes. "The doctor laughed at me. I kept going back and had to force them to run tests. They would take one look at me and say, 'There's nothing wrong with you. Get out of here.'"

"What were the results of the tests?" I ask Jeff.

"They were all normal. But I knew something was wrong. I mean, I'd get up and ache like hell all over. My joints, my muscles — I could hardly move. But every time they did the tests, they'd tell me there was nothing wrong. So I started doing my own research. I had to."

"What did you find out?"

"I started learning about my lab tests and what they meant. I started reading as much as I could. After a while, I knew more about the labs than some of the doctors. So I'd question them. My thyroid test came back low but inside the lab range for normal. The doctor said I was fine, so I asked him, 'Don't you think this is a little too low for a young guy like me?'

"What did he say?"

PRINCIPLE 5: CHANNEL CREATIVITY | 157

Jeff laughs. "He got angry. He tried to justify his answer and kept telling me, 'It's still normal.' So in the end, I had to do something for myself. I packed up the car and told my family I had to leave for Arizona. I drove 3,000 miles just so I could move my body again. And I kept trying to work on my health in every way possible. I did more research until I found out that I might have Lyme disease. And that's what I have; third stage. Doctors don't seem to know how to get the root cause of our problems as patients.

"That's when I decided to become a behavioral coach. I love helping people find their way to health, just like I did. I introduce them to the health practitioners who can really help them and are willing to collaborate with their doctors. If their doctors write them off, I tell them to find other docs who are willing to work for them, not vice versa. I'm at the center of their health networks. I don't know how you feel about that as a conventional doc, but that's what I do."

The Wheel of Health Manifestation™

Recall question Number 6 on the quick exercise you did at the beginning of this chapter: *Who is the most important person in your health network?* What is your answer to this question?

At the center of your health network is you! You are the most important provider of your health. Your doctor should not be at the center of this new medical model, making all the decisions for you and telling you who to see and what to do. Your conventional doctor should be placed at the periphery of your network and have the humility to collaborate fully with the other providers you choose. If your doctor disagrees with their advice, you need to reawaken your curiosity. You must learn more about why he or she disagrees. Don't be afraid to question your doctor. Are they saying things because of their own fears, egos, or judgments?

Take a step back and see the bigger picture. Don't allow the old programs of an outdated healthcare system to block your pathways to health and healing. There are many ways we can heal as humans; not all of them are currently explainable by modern science. But as long as they don't cause harm and are beneficial, all doctors and patients should embrace them.

Conventional medicine, of course, has much to offer. There's a basic standard of care which has proven to be more beneficial than harmful with many diseases. But conventional medicine doesn't have all the answers. It's only one small part of a much larger picture. And you, in the end, ultimately have personal choice.

The following image represents your personal health network, the one you will create for yourself. It's called The Wheel of Health Manifestation. This is your personalized provider and practitioner network, one that's not dished up to you by your health insurance company like yesterday's leftovers! *You* are at the very center of this network. And you will be the captain of your own journey to health.

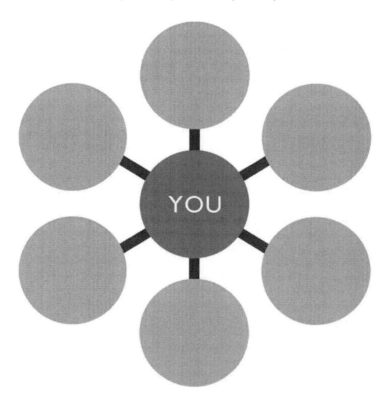

I invite you to fill in each of the circles with the names of the providers you listed earlier in this chapter. What do you think? Are there some changes you might want to make as you proceed with this new perspective in mind?

PRINCIPLE 5: CHANNEL CREATIVITY | 159

Now I'd like to take a moment to share with you my own personal Wheel of Health Manifestation. These are the actual health providers I have seen who have helped me to heal emotionally, physically, mentally, spiritually, and financially.

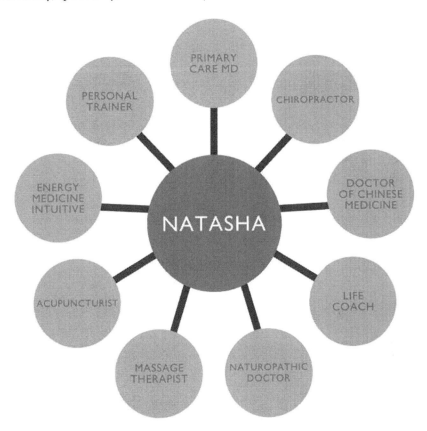

The Future's Not So Bright

The average life expectancy in the United States is currently about 78 years. This is an amazing thing. But if we take a closer look at who's living well into their 80s and 90s, we'll find that it's the people who were born and grew up in an era without health insurance. They, for the most part, did not have managed care networks. They did not even have Medicare programs. They did not pay so much money for outside parties to take care of them. They expected to take care of themselves, and so they did.

160 | THE 7 PRINCIPLES OF HEALTH

Today, we have an overweight and obesity rate greater than 73 percent in adults and better than 53 percent in our pediatric population. Even our dogs and cats are fat. We have epidemics of diabetes, heart disease, joint disease, cancer, mental illness, and many others. The money we put into cures has a bottomless pit. All this has come about in the age of health insurance, great technological advances, and pharmaceuticals that promise to keep us healthy. If we keep going the way we are, paying the government and health insurance to take care of us, coughing up money for drugs and procedures to fix us, do we really believe that our generation or the next will live well into their 80s, 90s, and beyond? And if, by chance, they do, will they live well?

Do you want to be a modern-day statistic? Do you want to wait for America's health system to change or wait for The Current Health Paradigm to shift? Or do you want something more for yourself, right here and right now?

The Health Integration Manager™ (H.I.M.)

Remember my friend Jeff? He said he was interested in helping patients navigate the complex medical system by becoming their health advocate. He's interested in helping them choose the right providers to guide them to health and empowering them to get rid of the ones who are keeping them sick. He wants to spend time coaching them on their behaviors as they relate to diet and exercise and supporting them through the tough times. He'd like to cheer them on and make sure they become the best they could ever be, helping them enjoy life to the fullest, no matter what their medical diagnoses.

Pastor John, Allison, Patricia, Don, Lyn, and many others have had to navigate their health on their own, often flying in the face of the authoritarian, negative attitudes of the medical profession. Wouldn't it be nice if we could all have a friend like Jeff to be with us in the center of our health network, supporting us along our journey to health?

A *Health Integration Manager (H.I.M.)* does exactly that. He or she helps with one of the critical components to our success in managing and even reversing disease: our behaviors. We all go through good times and bad times. So it's going to be vitally important to learn from the negative behaviors that contribute to our illness in order to find

PRINCIPLE 5: CHANNEL CREATIVITY | 161

health. And as we've already discussed, doctors are simply not equipped to help us manage — or change — these behaviors. They do not have the time, the training, or even necessarily the interest. They have been trained in their niche markets, and it's perfectly okay for them to remain in those niches, as long as we don't assume they understand everything about our bodies, minds, and spirits. They know a lot, but they do not know everything.

> *"Life deals you a lot of lessons; some people learn from it, some people don't."*
>
> **— Brett Favre**

What we need are allies who can help us create networks of alternate providers who are experts in their niches, too. That way we can benefit from the best of all worlds. We need someone who can help us coordinate the information from each of these experts and even interpret some of it. Sometimes we just need a shoulder to cry on or a hand to hold or someone to cheer us on. There's just not enough of that in a disease-based system that's focused on death, injury, illness, and dying, rather than the encouraging words of optimal health.

At the time of this writing, the certification program for the *Health Integration Manager* is just being launched. Sadly, in our current medical system, there isn't a coordinated plan to have someone like a H.I.M. work with patients at the center of their personalized networks. But don't despair! Help is on the way.

Sign up for our eNewsletter and visit us at health-conscious.org regularly to be the first to know when our certification program for the *Health Integration Manager* is launched! There will also be a lot of information to help you change your viewpoint, develop healthful practices, and see the biggest picture possible, which will then help you live a very different life than the one our healthcare system wants you to live. Who knows? You could be one of the very first team players in this exciting paradigm shift toward creating a new health model for our future.

162 | THE 7 PRINCIPLES OF HEALTH

YOUR INVITATION TO PRACTICE HEALTH

As you've been reading this book, you may have found yourself agreeing or disagreeing with some of the points I've made. That's perfectly all right; in fact, it is welcomed! Just as I'm advocating that you stand up against conventional medicine and its dogma, you can stand up against my ideas. You can help make them better! I invite you to take a moment to identify three areas I've presented so far in this book with which you agree and three things with which you disagree. Then, write down why you agree or disagree. Get it all out and be as honest as possible!

3 things with which I agree

1. _____

2. _____

3. _____

3 things with which I disagree

1. _____

2. _____

3. _____

You can visit us on Facebook, Twitter, LinkedIn, or Tumblr and hang out with us at health-conscious.org to post your comments. There is a lot more material for you to download and learn from as you move along your own journey to health. When we share as much information as possible in health, and teach each other from our stories and experiences, we all learn how to heal. We all find optimal health and live a fulfilled, happy life together!

CHAPTER EIGHT

Principle 6
Grow and Renew

"Dying is something we human beings do continuously,
not just at the end of our physical lives on this earth."

— **Elizabeth Kübler-Ross, M.D.** *(1926-2004)*
Swiss-American psychiatrist

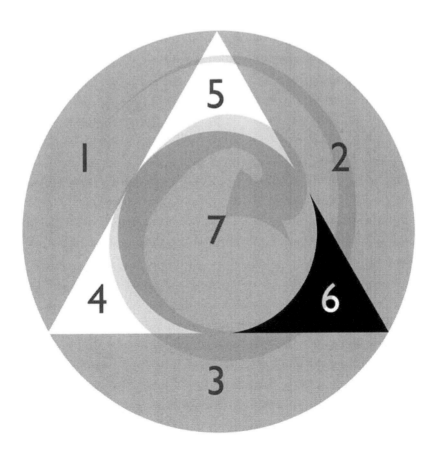

164 | THE 7 PRINCIPLES OF HEALTH

Natural law states that all living things change. Cycles are inherent in all forms of existence. In human life, we see this in the stages of conception, creation, growth and development, decline, and finally death. As Dan Millman, former Olympic gymnast and coach, states in his book, *The Life You Were Born to Live,* "The world of nature exists within a larger pattern of cycles, such as day and night and the passing of seasons ... all things happen in good time; everything has a time to rise, and a time to fall."

We can appreciate the dynamic nature of cycles in many other phenomena in our world. For example, nations and empires rise and fall; businesses are created, peak, and then decline; and celebrities are thrust into the limelight only to turn around and find they've become yesterday's news. Such is life. It ebbs and flows. It's continuous and dynamic. There is no constant except change. The concept of growth and renewal are an inescapable part of this natural law.

YOUR INVITATION TO PRACTICE HEALTH

Take a moment to try this exercise.

1. Find a few old photographs of yourself, spanning the last ten years or so. Lay them out next to each other in chronological order (oldest picture to most recent). Use the following approximate time periods: ten years, five years, three years, two years, one year ago, and today, if possible.

2. As you gaze at the pictures, pay attention to the words that come to mind. Write those words down on the following table.

3. To help organize your thoughts, you may want to associate your words with each of *The 5 Components of Total Health* listed across the top.

Number of Years Ago	Physical	Mental	Emotional	Spiritual	Financial
10					
5					
3					
2					
1					
Today					

166 | THE 7 PRINCIPLES OF HEALTH

4. Next, take a moment to read aloud the words you recorded on this table. What are some of your thoughts about the words you chose? Can you see that you've changed over time? How would you describe your changes as it applies to each of the different categories?

_____

_____

_____

_____

Ironically, when it comes to health and healthcare, the basic concept of growth and renewal has not been incorporated into clinical examinations, testing, or even the medical system. Somehow, in the context of medicine, we seem to have separated ourselves from natural law. You may be wondering what I mean by this. Let's examine this statement a little further.

If we take a look at the modern medical standard, the checkup examination, we find that it doesn't make sense when we think about it. The idea of a health check goes against our very nature of growth and renewal as living beings, because this type of exam is not representative of our state of health and doesn't really tell us if we are "in health" or healthy. It simply tells us that we do or don't have disease.

There are two key reasons for this: (1) the checkup as an examination tool is static or stationary; it's simply a series of snapshots in time, just like your photographs, and is not representative of the dynamic, continuous nature of human beings; and (2) the checkup is focused on screening for disease and is therefore not health-oriented.

The problem with the checkup does not lie with you and I, the patients and doctors. It occurs because our medical model is flawed. Take a minute to recall the earlier diagram of a patient and his or her relationship to the current healthcare system.

PRINCIPLE 6: GROW AND RENEW | 167

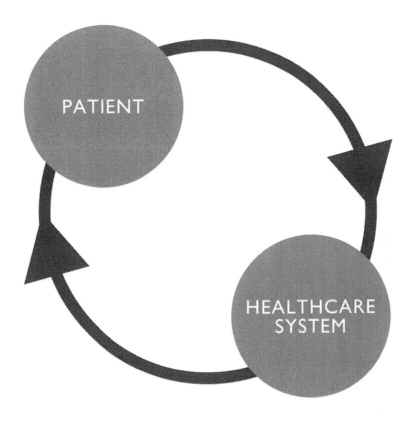

You and I, as patients, are not separate from our medical system, nor can we be separated from it. If there is a flaw in the way we've modeled things in the system, the same flaw will show up in us as patients. For example, say an architect creates a model of a house on the computer but forgets to insert a supporting wall in his diagram. What do you think the builders will do? They'll probably follow his plan, and the house will likely collapse because the supporting wall was vital to its construction. Likewise, in medicine, when we've modeled a healthcare system on static and disease-focused checkups and tests, we are guaranteed to become exactly that which we've created.

Our modern healthcare model is inconsistent with natural law for two reasons: (1) the health check (i.e., checkup) is a key component to determine the stats of our health but is a *static* exam; and (2) the checkup is doctor-centric (keeps a doctor at the center of the model), and since doctors are trained in disease by the system and not health, the exam cannot help but be disease focused rather than health focused.

If our individual examinations throughout the course of our lives are static and disease focused, and our medical system is modeled on disease and static testing, what is the only thing we can become?

●

"Mr. Jones, I see you're here because of a cough. But you've listed all these heart medications on your history form. How long have you been on them?"

"A few months now," Mr. Jones tells me. "I was fine until I saw the cardiologist," he laughs.

"What do you mean?"

"Well, I went in for a regular heart checkup, you know, from the referral my primary care doctor gave me. I wasn't having any problems, just wanted to get checked out, you know. He did a whole lot of tests and then sent me home with a clean bill of health. A couple days later, I found myself in the hospital having a heart attack."

The Flipbook Medical Exam

We can think of static checkups and disease-focused "health" examinations in medicine as similar to a flipbook of 300 blank pages. Imagine that an artist has drawn a series of stick figures on each page. He positions the stick figure slightly differently in each of the 300 different page views. For example, he might draw the stick figure's arm parallel to its body on one page and then on the next, the stick figure's arm might be slightly higher. As we advance the pages, we see that the stick figure's arm rises higher on each picture until 10 pages later, the arm is at 90 degrees to the stick figure's body.

PRINCIPLE 6: GROW AND RENEW | 169

Now imagine you turn each of the 300 pages slowly, one at a time. You gaze at each picture for several seconds. What will the stick figure look like to you? It will look like a stick figure!

This time, flip the pages of the book rapidly in succession and watch the artist's drawing. If he's worth his salt, his stick figure drawing will appear to move! It will look as though Mr. Stick is dancing or waving at us. In the old days, this is how Saturday morning cartoons were made. But we, as kids, believed that the characters could actually move on their own.

The Saturday morning cartoons represent the way our medical system was set up. When you book a health checkup with your doctor, he or she will examine you and then send you for a bunch of tests to screen for disease. They might send you for a panel of blood work, order an x-ray or colonoscopy, or perform any number of the increasing myriad of tests we have available at our fingertips today, thanks to advanced technology. But what does each of these tests show?

After your doctor gets the results back from all your tests, he or she reviews them. If they're all negative, he or she will conclude that you don't have a disease and are healthy. You then return home, believing that you are in good health. But is that necessarily true, as seen with Mr. Jones in the example above?

Let's say we took one of those tests your doctor had ordered, and stared at it, just like tearing a page out of our flipbook. What would we see? Would that test result represent you as a dynamic, continuous, integrated, functional human being? Or would it show the past result of a static test your doctor had ordered a few days ago?

The series of tests we put patients through during the course of their growth and development gives us a close approximation of their state of disease. They do not, however, give us a picture of their state of health. The absence of disease does not equal the presence of health. Similarly, a series of snapshots does not represent a dynamic, multidimensional view of us as living systems.

170 | THE 7 PRINCIPLES OF HEALTH

YOUR INVITATION TO PRACTICE HEALTH

I invite you to try this next exercise.

1. Recall the table you completed earlier in this chapter that contains the descriptions of how you've changed over time.

2. For this exercise, recall any doctors' visits you may have had over the years in which you were diagnosed with medical conditions. For example, maybe your doctor said you were hypertensive about three years ago and put you on medication. This example has been entered into the accompanying table.

3. Try and keep your "diagnoses" or problems in their respective categories. You may think the financial category does not represent a disease condition. But recent global economic and healthcare issues have created tremendous anxiety and stress in our personal lives. These are disease-labels, the same as the labels a doctor gives you (e.g., diabetes, heart disease, etc.) and should be approached in the same way. You and I know that the stress caused by money issues can and does affect our ability to find optimal health in the other areas. When it comes to total health, each of the separate categories listed has equal weight. They all affect our total health in very profound ways, regardless of the messaging inherent in our current medical paradigm.

Number of Years Ago	Physical	Mental	Emotional	Spiritual	Financial
10			EXAMPLE: Depression		
5					EXAMPLE: Mortgage Default
3	EXAMPLE: High BP				
2					
1					
Today					

172 | THE 7 PRINCIPLES OF HEALTH

4. What do you think of your new diseases and problems table? Do you see any patterns showing up that you hadn't noticed before? Do you see any imbalances showing up in one or more of the categories listed?

The 5 Components of Total Health

The definition of health is the creation of a balanced state in all aspects of our lives. We know that our environment is a key factor in our health. In fact, research detailed by cell biologist Dr. Bruce Lipton in his book, *The Biology of Belief*, demonstrates that our environment can play a much greater role in our health than our genetics. This environment includes not only physical, mental, and emotional components, but financial and spiritual ones, as well.

Unfortunately, modern medicine has focused mainly on disease, as we are coming to understand. We have become so super-specialized and intent on curing specific disease states that we've forgotten about the integrated human being. Each specialist focuses his or her expertise on specific cures or treatments, and thereby specific illnesses. If something else is going on in a patient's life, like stress or anxiety, the patient is quickly referred to another specialist.

Standard treatment by that next specialist (e.g., psychiatrist or psychologist) would likely be to prescribe an anti-anxiety or antidepressant drug, similar to Hope's case at the beginning of this book. But what if these unbalanced emotional states were the cause of imbalance in other key components of total health? Is it reasonable to say that these chronic emotional states can and do lead to physical manifestations of diseases such as very real heart attacks, hypertension, and strokes? Could it be that these unbalanced emotional states cause chronic inflammation in our bodies and an excess of damaging hormones like cortisol, which lead to inflammation in our blood vessels and cellular environments? Could this chronic inflammation in our bodies lead to the very cancers which subspecialists are so intent on curing in isolation, often forgetting to even consider the root causes of disease? More often than we may realize — and certainly more often than we've been taught — diseases are easily correctible through behavior and environmental changes, not through modern medicines and technology.

PRINCIPLE 6: GROW AND RENEW | 173

Because of such a narrow focus on disease, health management and disease treatment has been geared toward fixes and cures, rather than on determining the root causes or seeking optimal health balance. What if a health provider were to integrate our problems by taking a big picture view of all of *The 5 Components of Total Health*, thereby pointing us in directions that would truly help us heal?

Recall my personal trainer's friend who had breast cancer and decided to skip Timothy Brantley's healthy eating book, *The Cure*, and "go the medical route." If we understood the big picture, we would never believe that toxic drugs are better for our health than nutritious food. We would understand that addressing what we put into our bodies (e.g., food, air, and water) and on our skin (e.g., chemicals and toxins) also determines our state of health. We would understand that addressing our emotional balance, pre- and post-disease, is crucial to healing as multidimensional human beings who are continuously growing and renewing. We would then approach health from a very different point of view.

The following diagram illustrates once again how *The 5 Components of Total Health* are related.

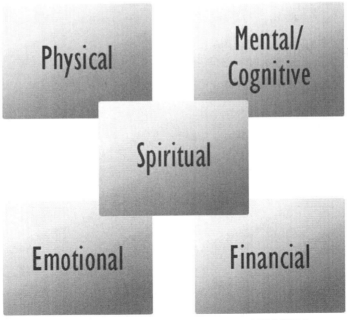

FIVE COMPONENTS OF TOTAL HEALTH

174 | **THE 7 PRINCIPLES OF HEALTH**

When we are out of balance in any one of these five components, we are diseased. Like you and I as the patient and doctor, and our relationship to our medical system, each one affects the others. A problem in one area creates a problem in the others. This is because we are integrated with our medical system, just as we are integrated as human beings, and not a set of separate parts that can be fixed in isolation. When one part is sick, the entire system is sick.

In the next section, we will return to some of the statements presented at the beginning of this book and explore what we think of them now that we're beginning to see things from a different perspective.

The Medical Checkup

Consider the following statements again.

1. Humans (we) are separate from the Universe.

2. Humans (we) are integrated with our Universe.

What do you think of their meaning now? How about these?

1. I must be cured from disease (separated).

2. My body has an innate capacity to heal (integrated).

Which perspective do you now hold as more representative of the way you want to see things?

The Medical System

1. "Medicine treats disease."

2. "Health reverses disease."

What do you think of these statements? As we consider a different way of seeing things, it becomes apparent that the more we continue to search for and create medicines to fix diseases, the less health we will have. When we begin to practice health at every opportunity and place our focus squarely on health, not disease, our behaviors change. These balanced actions as they pertain to each of *The 5 Components of Total Health* will lead to total health.

PRINCIPLE 6: GROW AND RENEW | 175

Consider the following statements as well.

1. "The doctor is the center of medicine." [DOCTOR-CENTRIC]

2. "You are the center of health." [INDIVIDUAL OR PATIENT-CENTRIC]

Would you now agree that the more a disease-oriented professional is placed at the center of our healthcare, the less health we will find, simply because that professional has spent a lifetime working within the minute details of disease, and can only think, act, prescribe and communicate from a disease-focused perspective?

We must become the drivers of our own health and create networks of health practitioners around us who can truly guide us to health. Yes, we must remove the physician from the center of The Wheel of Health Manifestation and put him or her at the periphery, along with many other practitioners of equal or greater value to us in our health practice. The health system fails to understand that physicians are niche market professionals in disease. Doctors are disease experts, not health experts. And it's neither possible nor necessary for all doctors to suddenly learn about total health. In fact, the most they could do would be to superficially advise you about diet and exercise, for no other reason than because they have spent years and years focused in disease. And we need them to remain focused on disease, to help provide the expert advice at which they are uniquely skilled. We will always need doctors in our networks; there's no doubt about that. Medicine has come too far to discard their expertise entirely. We just don't need them to dictate *all* aspects of our health anymore. We cannot expect doctors to lead us to health when their paradigms begin with disease.

So what's the answer, then? It lies in doctors' willingness to relinquish ego and judgment, to allow you, the patient, to make the final decision and to truly share the practice of health with many other experts who have already been practicing health much longer than we have. It lies in our willingness to open our minds and see something different than what we've been told to see.

176 | THE 7 PRINCIPLES OF HEALTH

YOUR INVITATION TO PRACTICE HEALTH

Now, let's try one more exercise.

Recall the tables you filled out earlier in this chapter. The first one shows the different ways in which you've changed over the years. The second one takes a look at your disease diagnoses or problems in each of the five categories. This time, let's focus exclusively on health actions. A health action is a practice or habit that is health oriented. Taking medication for high blood pressure is not a health action. It is a disease-focused action to prevent disease. What we want to focus on are those things which are done as health practice, not because you've got a disease. For example, following a nutritional plan, getting regular exercise, losing weight and practicing Tai Chi are health-oriented actions, regardless of disease.

1. Try and think of as many health actions which fit in each of *The 5 Components of Total Health*. List those which you have engaged in longer than one year and have led to changes in the way you live your life. For example, if you began a regular yoga practice 5 years ago and still practice today, write that down under "PHYSICAL." As another example, if you began working with an energy medicine practitioner and have learned how to let go of your childhood traumas, write that down under EMOTIONAL or SPIRITUAL health changes. If you worked with a financial planner and came up with a correction plan for your personal debt ratio, put that under FINANCIAL health. Some of your health actions may apply to more than one category. That's fantastic! That's just the way it should be. Health is multidimensional, just like what we are.

Number of Years Ago	Physical	Mental	Emotional	Spiritual	Financial
10					
5	EXAMPLE: Yoga Practice				
3			EXAMPLE: Energy Medicine		
2					
1					EXAMPLE: Financial Planner
Today					

178 | THE 7 PRINCIPLES OF HEALTH

2. Now take some time to review your notes. Compare this health-oriented action table with the previous one where you wrote down your disease-oriented actions. What do you think? Did you notice anything interesting? Do you feel differently about health practice versus disease or medical practice, now that you've come this far?

A Quick Summary of The 7 Principles of Health

Recall *The 7 Principles* we've learned so far. In order to first create in our minds a new approach to self-driven healthcare, we need to begin immediately with Principle 1, *Be Present*.

As you've been able to see, our medical system and all its delivery components — doctors, hospitals, health insurance, lawyers, pharmaceutical companies, and the government — are set up to see only one way of doing things. That way is highly disease focused. If we're going to remap our brains for health, we'll first need to stop all the noise, eliminate distraction, and learn how to focus on health. We'll need to empower ourselves. One way of doing this is through quiet meditation, beginning with just one minute a day and increasing from there. In the gap of silence, like our earlier AED example, we can reconfigure our thoughts and re-program our messages.

Next, we needed to understand our medical system and how it affects each of us. In Principle 2, we learned how to **Become Aware**. There is plenty of information about health and health statistics out there. Being aware of who is generating that information and where their self-interest lies helps us understand whether the information they provide will be good for our health or not.

In Principle 3, *Be Health*, we created our Personal Health Mantra to remind us every day that we all have an innate capacity to heal. These health mantras help us direct our old messages away from disease thoughts and toward health, regardless of any labels we may already have received from the current conventional health system. We realized that we were always in health. We were designed in every instance to *Be Health*.

In Principle 4, we learned to **Reawaken Curiosity** by researching more about health without the distraction of disease, fear, ego, or judg-

PRINCIPLE 6: GROW AND RENEW | 179

ment. We learned how to keep our minds open and set aside those messages which would not serve us well on our journey to health. We learned that health requires integration every day and that it can be found by adding alternative modalities to conventional medical practice in a very balanced way. We learned that we didn't have to feel embarrassed about those who were helping us because we were simply learning more about their practice, rather than passing judgment.

In Principle 5, *Channel Creativity*, we learned to add our favorite providers to our personal health networks. Suddenly, we found ourselves at the center of our own health creation, able to make decisions for ourselves. We began to embrace the concept of real health and leave disease, fear, and disempowerment far behind.

Finally, in this chapter, we learned the natural law of cycles. In Principle 6, *Grow and Renew*, we learned that life is continuous. It changes every moment. It is integrated. We learned that we cannot separate ourselves from life because we are, in fact, life. And we learned that when we use a static medical model and keep disease-focused practice at its center, we become what we've practiced. But when we understand that health is found through continuous change and collaboration, we become healthy.

Perhaps it seems like this is all going to be very difficult to accomplish, especially with such well-entrenched external stakeholders in modern medicine needing to keep us focused on out-dated disease ideas and concepts. But despite this, we each have a wonderful opportunity to change, especially as we enter a new era of consciousness in our human existence. In his book, *The Whole Brain Path to Peace*, philosopher James Olson states that we can alter our perspectives by switching from left-brain to right-brain dominance and then merging the two to create a very different way of thinking, as well as a more productive and fulfilled life. Nowhere is this concept more evident than in medicine, which seems to be the last bastion of left-brain dominance. By accepting and utilizing a greater portion of our total brain capacity, we can all become much, much healthier and lead happier, more fulfilled lives.

Those individuals who are able to see different paradigms in healthcare are the ones who will be able to truly balance the different disciplines of medicine and health practice. They will open themselves to their inner sources of healing. Richard Gerber, M.D., says in his book, *A Practical Guide to Vibrational Medicine*:

> While disease is generally seen as a negative experience, the potential for transformation exists in all illness, not only for sick individuals but also for those around them as well. The outcome depends upon how those individuals choose to deal with that illness and how they use their experience to relate to others.

Hopefully this book has been able to show that you have choice in every aspect of your life, including your health.

A New Health Model

In this section, we will examine how to create a new model of health-care delivery and a new health monitoring exam that replaces the "checkup."

We'll always need to be screened for disease in some way or another. There's no doubt that modern medicine has come a long way and has found many miraculous cures. It's our intention — our narrow focus on excluding disease first as representative of our health status — that we need to change.

As we've seen by now, it's not possible to separate ourselves as patients from our medical system. Since we currently have a very doctor-centric medical model, we currently believe that doctors must make changes first, and then we will follow all their advice. We may also erroneously look to external stakeholders and wait for them to change. But what have we learned? Who is the only person who can change you? Relying on a government mandate that we purchase health or be punished will never work for all people or over the long term.

Many doctors know that their patients are desperately searching for something different to help them, and that they're driving their own care, largely because of skyrocketing costs. But some experts are advising that in order to keep up with the health trends which you, the patient, are demanding, doctors should be the ones to learn more about nutrition and health practice in medical school. Doctors should be the ones to direct you toward health.

PRINCIPLE 6: GROW AND RENEW | 181

What's the problem with this proposal? For a moment, let's set aside the time it takes to educate doctors to become experts in disease, somewhere in the ballpark of 12 to 15 years, plus all the additional time it takes to keep up with advancing treatments and technology in their careers. Let's set aside the time it will take to reeducate an entirely new generation of young doctors to become experts in disease and health practice. We'll also have to put aside the layers and layers of bureaucracy and extensive time it will take to morph

> *"The greater the ignorance, the greater the dogmatism."*
>
> — **Sir William Osler**

into a health-oriented paradigm like the one we've been discussing in this book, especially since it's taken America more than 100 years to realize that serious health reform is necessary for its citizens. We'll leave aside the external stakeholders who will, no doubt, viciously fight any change that disturbs their billions-per-quarter profits. We'll also have to let go of the fact that doctors are in critically short supply, aging and burning out rapidly from their professions, with fewer and fewer next-generation replacements enrolling in medical schools. And finally, we'll have to ignore the fact that changing a doctor's practice habits will take some 17 to 20 years to become the new standard of care.

Does it make more sense for you to wait, or to change yourself first, finding your own way to optimal health despite these external hurdles? Isn't it possible to pay much less for your personal healthcare by simply changing the way *you* see things?

Of course it is! But no one said it was going to be easy. So how can you start right now to ensure that you find your way to cost-effective health by using your new perspective? How can you be the driving force to change healthcare for yourself and your nation?

You are already doing it! You've been creating your own health networks inside the old disease-focused medical model. You've been searching for other answers. You've been taking a critical look at what doctors are telling you and questioning whether it's going to be right for you. And, you have been out there desperately searching for answers.

Consumers currently drive the complementary and alternative health (CAM) markets. They pay these expenses out of pocket, money

182 | THE 7 PRINCIPLES OF HEALTH

that is outside of disease-care cost. In the 10 years from 1997 to 2007, this market grew from $27 billion to $33.9 billion.[39] If you asked most conventional doctors 10 years ago — and even some today — if acupuncture should be considered a health practice, they would have said no. But what's our opinion today? Many practices are finally integrating both complementary and alternative treatments along with conventional medicine, realizing that you, the consumer, are the experts in your own health.

So the creation of a new medical model is already happening! You are creating it, and you've done so by following *The 7 Principles of Health* as outlined in this book, although you may not have been aware you were doing it. All you need now is a *Health Integration Manager* who will essentially take your hand as you navigate your personal health network (The Wheel of Health Manifestation) and seek expert consultation in many different fields. By doing so, you will find longevity, youth, and excellent health. You will be able to heal, as necessary.

The final struggle will come down to the way you view things, as we've said throughout this book. Since The Current Health Paradigm is heavily doctor-centric, patients still look to doctors to be the experts in health. But remember, they are not. Even with a vast amount of training over many years, they are not health experts. They are disease experts.

Who out there is already trained in aspects of health, already passionately niched in each of their areas of expertise, and already cost effective? Many physicians may fear that they will now be saddled with the burden of learning disease medicine, health practice, alternative practice, business, bureaucracy, nutritional counseling, psychological counseling, and manipulative medicine. But why do doctors have to know and do it all? Can we take a page from our business compatriots who seem to have figured things out much more quickly than we have in medicine?

Many businesses create niche markets in which they become experts. They then network and collaborate with other businesspeople

---

[39]Costs of Complementary and Alternative Medicine, July 30 2009, National Health Statistics Reports Number 18, Centers for Disease Control. Accessed online at http://www.cdc.gov/nchs/data/nhsr/nhsr018.pdf.

PRINCIPLE 6: GROW AND RENEW | 183

to provide resources and referrals to those in other areas of expertise. They create arrangements similar to the Wheel of Health Manifestation. Is it absolutely necessary for doctors to stay at the center of our health model, multitasking their way to insanity and burning out by trying to be disease, business, and health experts, or would it be much more efficient to create networks and collaborate?

Ego and judgment are sure to step in at this point. The health practice model I'm describing moves the doctor to the periphery of your healthcare. The disease-focused doctor becomes more of a niche expert in disease, while collaborating with nutritionists, energy medicine healers, acupuncturists, herbalists, holistic practitioners — and yes, even psychics, mediums, clairvoyants, and hypnotists! This type of network is already being created by many, many people who understand *The 5 Components of Total Health*. No single opinion is superior to another, except yours. This is your health network and your health plan, so you can invite into it anyone whose advice seems to work for you.

This medical model is more representative of a perspective that begins with health first. It uses the expertise of a vast array of practitioners from all sides of the medical spectrum and incorporates them into a truly collaborative framework, with you at the center. In this model, you have become fully empowered to make your own choices, based on each expert's advice.

This medical model is also dynamic and integrated. There is no longer a checkup at the center of the health system. It's more of a health monitoring system, a continual dynamic process that recognizes and incorporates natural law. You will likely still have checkups that screen for disease, but you will also make many other appointments in your health practice, as opposed to the current disease practice. For example, regular massage and meditation, energy healing or bodywork can help you heal from an integrated, multidimensional perspective. Regular acupuncture treatments can calm anxiety and stress, reducing the need for expensive, toxic antidepressant medications. Fitness and nutrition experts can help find body movements that are just right for your body, not for some celebrity whose job it is to stay ultra-fit. The doctor no longer has to preach "diet and exercise." These words will now have deep meaning for you because you will understand health practice.

184 | THE 7 PRINCIPLES OF HEALTH

So as you can see, by incorporating *The 7 Principles of Health*, *The 5 Disciplines of Health Practice*, *The 7 Requirements for Health Practice*, and by balancing *The 5 Components of Total Health*, you will *Be Health*, in every sense of the word.

And the only way to begin is to start right now.

Creating a New Baseline

There's one aspect of our current health paradigm we've yet to mention. That's the idea of some kind of a "test" that can diagnose us as integrated, energetic beings and provide a complete picture of our health in real time. As we've mentioned, current medical testing is essentially a series of snapshots taken over time. They're like the flipbook with its stick figure cartoons drawn on each page. Medical tests can be predictive of future probabilities, but they cannot predict outcomes with 100 percent certainty. As we've seen through the amazing stories in this book, we can use the new model to create our own outcomes for ourselves, regardless of scientific prediction, simply by changing our viewpoint.

Scientists and medical researchers are interested in discovering such a predictive health test. Some doctors, such as Dr. David Agus in his book, *The End of Illness*, say a field called proteonomics[40] will offer this future test. Unfortunately, however, machines that analyze our blood, determine our predisposition to disease, or evaluate our current state of nutrition are still unable to measure key components of our natural state. These scientific tests for which we continue to search are unable to take into account the degree to which our emotional, cognitive, and mental states affect our physical state. They are still static tests, and therefore cannot give us a complete picture of our total health.

The funny thing is that in science, we're always searching for a machine to do our bidding. As a doctor, I know we'd all love to have a machine that could give us an instantaneous dynamic view of our patients, right down to any preexisting diseases they might be harboring in their energetic fields. But when I look at things from a different perspective and begin to really think outside the boxes we have

---

[40]Proteonomics is the study of proteins that are made by the genes in the body.

PRINCIPLE 6: GROW AND RENEW | 185

constructed in medicine, I realize that we seem to be searching in the wrong place. We're not going to find what we're looking for from a machine. What we're looking for is right here in front of us, if we'd take the time to open our eyes and begin to think differently.

Machines are wonderful things. But, nothing is more miraculous than a human being. So the device medicine should be searching for to diagnose true and complete health is another human being, one who has intuitive energetic capabilities and can see the dynamic nature of our existence in total integration. There are people who can and do read energy fields, diagnose, and help heal — without drugs, pills, tests, or other procedures. There are people who can sense disease in energetic fields before it manifests as a physical state in our bodies. These many different fields are well researched and discussed in Dr. Richard Gerber's book, *A Practical Guide to Vibrational Medicine*. If we were to utilize these folks for a primary diagnosis, then support their findings with science and technology, can you imagine the ways in which we could truly heal?

The interesting thing is, this work has already been done for many, many years. Individuals such as clairvoyant Carolyn Myss and Harvard trained neurosurgeon, Dr. Norman Shealy, have pioneered the field and can attest to its success. New areas of bioenergetic healing are also emerging. Many conventional doctors are already collaborating with intuitive healers and psychics to trace not only the origins of preexisting diseases embedded in our energetic fields, but also to help clear blockages to our life force or *qi*. The information and studies about these practitioners are widely available but not fully accepted by conventional medical practice, which controls our so-called health.

You, as patients, are already utilizing these practitioners and their capabilities as part of your personal health in growing numbers, according to the recent National Health Statistics Reports. But conventional medicine, as prescribed by the external stakeholders that comprise today's medical system, will have none of that alternative stuff at this point. When we put our eyes to the lenses of our microscopes and live in fear of those things we cannot yet fully explain with scientific evidence, ironically, we in medicine tend to forget that we are all human beings. We forget how truly advanced we all are as a species and how we all have these miraculous healing abilities. So, we fall back on

186 | **THE 7 PRINCIPLES OF HEALTH**

our left-sided, analytical brains that dominate society and today's medical system and we wind up searching for something far, far inferior in capacity and capability.

I would encourage you to read the work of Gerber, Shealy, Myss, and many, many others who know that integrated, energetic diagnosis is possible and evidence based. As you can see, it is possible to work from a very different paradigm in healthcare. It is possible to create a new medical model and a new "diagnostic test" to help detect problems in all *5 Components of Total Health*. It is possible to find health. And, it is possible to change our world. In the end, you will decide how to synthesize all this information for yourself, stand up to a disease-focused system that needs to keep you sick in order to function, and learn to truly heal without fear.

●

Do you remember Hope's story from the very beginning of this book? She was caught in the maze of our modern medical system, desperately searching for answers to her problems. She'd been bounced back and forth between specialists and a primary care doctor, each one repeating the same tests and procedures and writing different prescriptions. Every time she tried to take a new pill to treat a symptom, she experienced side effects that made her feel much worse. This prompted her to seek more medical care, but somehow, the more she tried to integrate her healthcare, the more fragmented her care became. In the end, she felt utterly hopeless.

What if Hope were able to get help from a healthcare system based on The New Health Paradigm presented in this book? Let's examine what could happen.

A Time for Hope

Hope is 27 years old. She feels depressed and has gained a lot of weight. She's having relationship troubles with her husband and kids and feels that the stress in her life is causing her world to spiral down into a dark hole.

According to The Wheel of Health Manifestation that Hope cre-

PRINCIPLE 6: GROW AND RENEW | 187

ated to support herself — her personal health network — she is at the center of her health model. In other words, she can and will make choices for her own health. She's not a doctor and she doesn't know exactly what is wrong, but instead of taking the backward approach of looking at the problem first or searching first for a disease label and then trying to fix things, she begins with the bigger picture in mind.

Instead of rushing to see her primary care physician, she first consults with her Health Integration Manager. The goal of her H.I.M. is not to replace a doctor's advice; he's there to help her navigate her personal network of health providers.

Hope's H.I.M. listens to her. He spends time with her. He provides initial emotional support and counseling, which help empower her to feel that she can find the answers she seeks. He then sets up an initial plan that includes regular visits for support and guidance over the next few months.

Next, Hope's H.I.M. tells her that she does need a doctor's advice to confirm or rule out a potential disease. Hope's primary care doctor is familiar with Eastern and Western medical practice and also is experienced in functional medicine. Functional medical practitioners are trained to look at integrated systems to see how they interact and affect the whole. They are not trained to search for the details of an isolated disease; neither do they seek to treat isolated symptoms or signs.

Hope sees her functional medicine primary care doctor who examines her and sends her for a few lab tests. He finds that although her thyroid is within the normal range for a standard disease lab, other more detailed panels of endocrine testing (T3, anti-thyroid antibodies, progesterone, estrogen, etc.) show that she is suffering from Hashimoto's thyroiditis, one of the most common forms of thyroid gland problems. The symptoms associated with this disease include depression, inability to lose weight, sluggishness, lack of energy, dry skin, menstrual disturbances, and muscle or joint aches and pains. Her functional medicine doctor advises her on a treatment plan to correct the root cause of her symptoms. He makes recommendations for the minimal synthetic prescriptions necessary and asks Hope's input on the medications and formulas she'd like to take. He also offers to support her with natural, plant-derived herbs and formulations.

Hope returns to her H.I.M. to discuss her progress. She tells him that she and her primary doctor are working on the medical part of

188 | THE 7 PRINCIPLES OF HEALTH

her problems. Her H.I.M. congratulates her and asks her if there are any other areas in her overall health plans she may want to work on at this point. Hope tells him that she wants to see a nutritionist to help her learn more about an anti-inflammatory diet. Since Hope has an autoimmune disease that's related to inflammation, this type of nourishment will help reduce some of her symptoms and make her feel better. Though she has been attending group nutrition sessions regularly and has learned a lot from them, she feels she could benefit from a more specific plan, now that her functional medicine doctor has made a diagnosis. Hope's H.I.M. tells her that's a great idea.

On her next visit to her functional medicine doctor, Hope tells him her symptoms are improved. Not only is her pain reduced, but her relationships with her family are happier, and work is better, too. She feels she could still do with some supportive counseling, so she engages the services of a psychologist.

Over the next few months, Hope continues to improve. She's corrected her nutrition and has also been seeing her personal fitness consultant who has her on a graduated program to health. Her trainer started Hope at a level that's just right for her, not a generic cookie-cutter standard. She's feeling better every day and joins a women-only social group where she's been able to get out and have fun. In addition, she's begun to incorporate massage therapy and acupuncture into her monthly treatment plans. Both practitioners are working with her underlying disease condition, but Hope has found that this bodywork has helped many of her symptoms, as well as her mental and emotional states of health.

During one of her massage sessions, Hope has flashes of her past during the session and breaks down into tears. Her massage therapist explains that she's having an emotional release. Her therapist suggests that she work with an energy medicine practitioner to see if clearing up some of those blockages to her emotional state can help.

When Hope works with the energy practitioner, she realizes that she was abused as a child, a memory she has suppressed for many years. Rather than face it head on, she developed a subconscious sense of self-loathing that had metaphorically manifested as an autoimmune disease. Her self-loathing had become a real, physical illness. Her body was trying to destroy itself with antibodies to its own tissues. Hope

PRINCIPLE 6: GROW AND RENEW | 189

worked with her energy medicine practitioner to begin releasing the tight grip on her past, thereby clearing the emotional and cognitive path for her to live a very different life in the future, one that is much more self-loving.

By the end of six months, Hope has lost about 50 pounds. She's no longer having relationship difficulties and she loves life. She loves herself enough to

> *"If you can dream it, you can do it."*
>
> — **Walt Disney**

make sure she has personal and social time, every day. She checks in regularly with her functional primary care doctor and her supportive counselors, but she finds she no longer needs such intense work to clear the earlier issues and challenges. She's hardly taking any medication and she feels the best she's felt in years. She reports back to her H.I.M. who smiles and tells her she's an amazing person.

And we all know that she is.

●

Does this sound like a science fiction movie, or fantasy novel? Is it so unreasonable to change our paradigms from the way we've always seen things in medicine to imagine possibilities of health and reconstruct our thoughts toward manifesting them in our lives?

All the elements for this New Health Paradigm model are already in place. There's actually not a lot of technical work necessary to accomplish it; the effort will involve stopping ourselves from being so afraid to stand up for our right to live a great life.

Divergent fields in both alternative and conventional medicine are growing, becoming well studied and acceptable to all. The pendulum toward balance in health is already swinging, largely driven by ordinary people like you and me, without the so-called expert authority of an archaic medical system which is often the last to embrace change. All that's left is to release the tight grip of those who want to keep you sick so you can change your paradigm.

The decision is up to you in the end. Which way do you choose to see things? Which paradigm do you now see? You alone have the power to choose the actions you take.

So, how will *you* choose to live before you die?

CHAPTER NINE

Principle 7
Heal, Change, and Thrive

"One of the essential qualities of the clinician is interest in humanity, for the secret of the care of the patient is in caring for the patient."
— Francis W. Peabody, M.D. *(1881-1927)*
Harvard-trained physician, researcher, and teacher

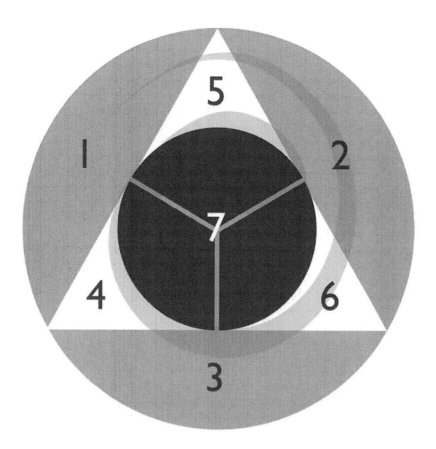

PRINCIPLE 7: HEAL, CHANGE, AND THRIVE | 191

"Hey, Doc, can you write me a letter?" Don's voice is on the other end of the telephone. He sounds weaker than I remember, and his voice is now laced with the tone of someone who's about to give up his fight. I know that tone of voice very well. "I'm flying to Alaska, for good," he continues. "It's the only way I'll be able to afford treatment. I need the letter so I can take my dog onto the airplane. It has to be for medical reasons."

"We don't normally do that in urgent care, Don," I say quietly.

"I know, Doc. But I can't afford another visit. I just can't."

"What are you going to do in Alaska?"

"They won't help me here. I have to go — there's this old pastor of mine. He's started a fund to help me out."

"What about state health insurance? What about your job?" I ask.

"Are you kidding? They won't cover me because my wife earns a few bucks more than their cut off. And I'm too sick to work. The insurance plan dropped me a long time ago; I haven't been covered for a couple of years now. Besides, what employer these days is going to pay for a liver transplant?"

"I'm sorry, Don." The silence between us is endless. His drawn face flashes in my mind, and I recall the way his eyes had dimmed as the months passed. "What do you need the letter to say?"

"My dog's name is Pug. Just write that Pug can accompany me on the airplane, that it's necessary for emotional support. That's what they want it to say."

"I'll leave it for you at the front desk, okay?"

"Thanks, Doc." Another endless silence stretches between us. "And, Doc, I want to thank you for all you've done."

"Take care of yourself, Don. Good luck." The phone clicks and inside of a second, he's gone.

Heal

Recall our heart attack victim from the beginning of the book. We left him strapped to the leads of an AED, the automated external defibrillator. The electrical current sent to depolarize his heart cells had effectively stopped them from beating.

Inside this gap, we hope our victim's body has had time to figure things out. We hope his heart cells have reset their internal pacemaker

192 | THE 7 PRINCIPLES OF HEALTH

function and will begin to beat again, this time together in a synchronous rhythm that will pump blood throughout his body, awaken him to consciousness, and allow him to live.

Similar to our victim, this book is like an AED. It has presented a different way of seeing things in health and healthcare, in ourselves, and within our medical system. And hopefully, it has served to reconfigure the thoughts that will lead to synchronous actions that are geared toward keeping our hearts beating strong, enabling us to live in health for a long time to come.

> *"It's never too late to be what you might have been."*
>
> — **George Eliot**

In Principle 7, we find that we can *Heal, Change, and Thrive.* After learning about Principles 1 through 6 and putting them into daily practice, or creating a habit, we have arrived at our big-picture goal: optimal health. Our process first began with a shift in our paradigm. We began to see things from a new perspective. Let's take a brief look at the path we've just traveled.

Reprinted on the following page is The Current Health Paradigm and The New Health Paradigm. Take a moment to review these words once again. What are some of your thoughts, now that you have almost completed this book? Take a moment to circle the words that seem to resonate well with you at this point.

PRINCIPLE 7: HEAL, CHANGE, AND THRIVE | 193

The Current Health Paradigm	The New Health Paradigm
Quick Fix	Long-term
Fragmented	Whole
Individualistic	Collective
Cure	Heal
Disease-oriented	Health
Mechanical	Energetic System
Polarized	Balanced
Victimization	Empowered
Paternalistic	Guide or Teacher
Mandate	Collaborative
Blame	Accountable
Judgment	Nonjudgmental
Myopic	Clear Vision
Unconscious	Conscious

When we begin to see things differently, we understand that in the context of health, death does not mean that we've failed — as patients or as doctors. We all have the power to heal. It's contained deep within our core, just as Principle 7 is diagramed inside the figure. This healing comes not only in physical form, but also in emotional, mental, spiritual, and financial components. As with Don in the previous story, some conditions are terminal. Medical science can offer no cure. We sometimes have to accept this. But Don's healing can and will come in the form of the strong community spirit he's about to return to that will help him live well, despite his terminal diagnosis. In this sense, Don has found optimal health.

Where have we failed Don in medicine? It doesn't lie in the fact that he'll die. That is a fate we all must accept. Our failure lies in the fact that we have not offered Don a chance to live. We allowed the construction of such a brutal system that primarily seeks to keep the individual as far from health as possible for the sake of profit, to focus our eyes on the pursuit of disease. This relentless pursuit has sickened us financially. From our financial imbalance, we have subsequently become emotionally, mentally, and physically imbalanced. And we are

194 | **THE 7 PRINCIPLES OF HEALTH**

now experiencing the final assault on our health in the form of our spiritual demise.

This is where we're headed. Unless we change our paradigms as individuals first, employing our ability to choose for ourselves in every health decision we make, and to think differently, as Einstein advised, no one else out there will ever be able to solve our problems, regardless of the promises they may make. Only when we learn to end the distraction and fear-mongering embedded deep in our society, stop the victimization and disempowerment, recognize the voices of ego and judgment, and make our own decisions as unique individuals, will we change and thrive. Our power to heal comes from our own life source, contained deep inside our beings. As we journey through life, we can learn exactly how to live well and enjoy every moment of every day, no matter who tells us otherwise.

YOUR INVITATION TO PRACTICE HEALTH

Let's take a moment to reflect on a few things as they relate to our personal quest for health.

1. Write down three personal health issues that you're worried about.

   a. _____

   b. _____

   c. _____

2. Write down three things that might stop you from changing those worries into opportunities or successes.

   a. _____

   b. _____

   c. _____

PRINCIPLE 7: HEAL, CHANGE, AND THRIVE | 195

3. Can you identify any instances where you might change the way you look at things and start from a different place or see a new perspective? Comment on that below.

_____

_____

_____

_____

Change

Change is often said to come from the inside-out. But change is also a very difficult thing for many of us to do. It's our natural tendency to want things to stay the same. And sometimes, we want things the same so we can keep complaining about them.

When it comes to health, our most precious asset, we seem to be stuck. Many of us realize that as we age, our old habits begin to catch up to us. We can't eat the same way we used to. We can't sit around and surf the Internet or watch T.V. the way we used to, and expect not to get fat. We can't continue to burn out in stressful jobs or careers that no longer hold meaning or passion. We seem to want change, but try as we might, we can't quite do it.

Why not? There are many things in healthcare to distract us from change. If we have the challenges of disease, we live from hospital to doctor's office to operating room. We shovel pills down our throats and try to keep our spirits high enough to make it to our next disease-focused doctor's appointments. We remain inside the box of disease. On the flip-side, if we're blessed with health, we spend more money from our personal savings to eat well, join gyms, lose weight, and accept a lower salary for work that we love to do, while still paying ridiculous amounts for escalating disease care. But the looming fear of health insurance costs and mandates erodes our endeavors. We never seem to get ahead in life or in health. We find that at the end of the day, after paying and paying for so-called healthcare, there's not enough energy or money left over for health practice.

Deep down, we're afraid that in the future, after squandering our money on someone else's diseases, there won't be enough left to fix

196 | THE 7 PRINCIPLES OF HEALTH

our own bodies when we're sick and broken, because we didn't take care of ourselves in this moment called now.

Change, then, from deep within our healthcare system will need to come from the outside-in, not in terms of waiting around for health insurance or the government to fix us, but in terms of clearly understanding the paradigm from which we operate. If we're all so busy, so stuck in the trivia and details of disease that we don't realize we're headed in the wrong direction, how can we ever expect to get where we really want to go? The only way to begin the change process is to stop, defibrillate, and **Be Present**. Once we've stopped the highly distracting input, we can begin our journey by orienting ourselves in a different direction — one that starts without fear. We can practice health instead of medicine.

Change in the context of our medical system starts from the outside-in, but on a personal level, it will always begin from the inside-out.

YOUR INVITATION TO PRACTICE HEALTH

Take a moment to try this quick exercise.

1. List the names of three people you care about deeply.

a. _____

b. _____

c. _____

2. If you could have anything at your fingertips with which to help each of these people, sort of like a genie in a bottle, how would you help him or her? Let your imagination run wild! Say your brother has been out of work for 18 months and you had a million dollars. How would you help him?

_____

_____

_____

PRINCIPLE 7: HEAL, CHANGE, AND THRIVE | 197

3. Why do you care about these people? Why do you want to help make a difference in their lives?

_____

_____

_____

4. If you can't think of any reasons, why do you think that might be?

_____

_____

_____

5. Now, take a short moment to consider the eulogy that will be read at your funeral. The three people you listed in Question 1 are attending. What would you want each of them to say about you and the life that you lead?

_____

_____

_____

Thrive

The most common answer to the question, "What do you want to do with your life?" seems to be, "I want to make a difference." The most common regret dying people seem to have is the feeling that they didn't have the courage to stand for what they believed in and knowing they were unwilling to take a risk doing what they might have done.

We have always contained the power to heal inside us. It just took some effort to widen the lens of our personal and collective viewpoints so we could see this. We needed to find a different roadmap.

As you can see in The *7 Principles of Health* diagram, Principle 7, *Heal, Change, and Thrive* is contained in its heart center.

We have worked our way toward change from the outside-in. We've learned a tremendous amount regarding the paradoxical messaging and programming that is contained inside our healthcare system and the way we have been taught to see things as doctors and as patients. We've learned how to tap into our innate source of healing and allow it to guide our clinical treatments and health plans. Now it's time to work our way from the inside-out and continue to change, not only ourselves, but also our world. Our goal as humans should be to do far more than barely survive as a species on Earth, resigning ourselves to eventually destroying our home planet and the sources of life through short-sighted ignorance, greed, and power. Our innate desire should be to thrive.

You First

The heart of Principle 7, *Heal, Change and Thrive*, is divided into three chambers, or pieces of pie. The first describes the individual, you and me. How have we healed? How have we changed?

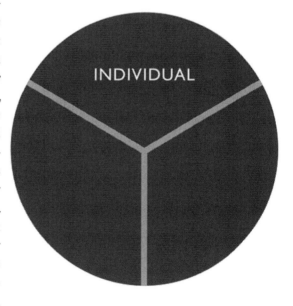

This part represents all we have learned in this book: the baby steps we've taken to navigate through *The 7 Principles of Health*, putting into practice what we've learned, and understanding the fundamental requirements we must embrace for lasting transformation. In small increments, just as the Serenity Prayer says, we've found the courage to stand up for the things we can change and the serenity to accept the things we cannot change. We've also found in this book the "wisdom to know the difference."

PRINCIPLE 7: HEAL, CHANGE, AND THRIVE | 199

We won't always be perfect beings. Inherent in our human nature is struggle, so we'll continue to struggle along the way, trying on new things, slipping backward now and again, but always moving forward. What we will discover along the way is that we've found the strength to argue for our beliefs, despite what others might say, and that we've taken a risk in defending our most precious home, our very lives.

> *"No man is an island."*
> — John Donne

Life is interdependent. We depend on our families, our neighbors, and our communities to get through life. Unfortunately, modern society has all but alienated us from each other, despite having the most advanced technology in history to keep us globally connected.

Community Second

The second piece of pie in Principle 7 represents our community. These communities are composed of the people with whom we interact every day, and those who are in positions of responsibility to create social order. They are local business owners, politicians, teachers, healthcare workers, students, developers, and many others. These are the people in your neighborhood.

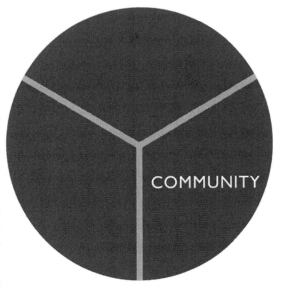

Our communities affect us and our families. The decisions of our community leaders also affect us. These decisions determine the types of food served in school cafeterias, the placement of power lines, the industries allowed into the area, and the enforcement of pollution controls to protect our environment. We cannot help but care about these decisions because these are the decisions that ultimately affect our health. These decisions determine the quality of the resources we require to stay alive.

By the time we've found our way to Principle 7, realizing we care about ourselves so profoundly that we seek high quality nourishment, air, water, and environments in which to live, we begin to profoundly care about our communities. To do anything other is simply impossible. Essentially, the needs of our bodies are determined not only by the things with which we choose to eat, drink, and surround ourselves, but also by the decisions our neighbors make, too. So developing a deep respect for our bodies through the practice of each of *The 7 Principles of Health* necessitates that we care about the changes affecting our neighborhoods, too. Ultimately, we become advocates for healing and changing not only ourselves, but our communities as well.

And Finally, Your World

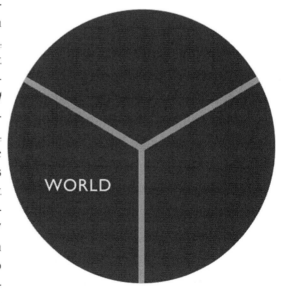

As individuals who depend on others and on whom others depend, we live our lives locally. However, when we embrace *The 7 Principles of Health*, we begin to realize that every thought, belief, and action we uphold also affects us as a global community. We are completely interdependent on the 7 billion other people on this planet. There is no escaping this reality, despite politics or wars. Whether or not we like it, there is only one kind of human being on this planet — and we're quickly destroying it.

PRINCIPLE 7: HEAL, CHANGE, AND THRIVE | 201

Are you more human than the destitute in Somalia because you have plenty of food on your table and they don't? Do you deserve to destroy another's land, food supplies, and air for all the diamonds or oil money can buy? As distant as they may seem, these actions only serve, in the end, to hurt us back here in our cozy homes. We can no longer separate ourselves from our globe and all the other souls on it.

Therefore, caring for our planet is the default position when it comes to caring for ourselves. We can't help it because we've found a new respect for every morsel we put into our bodies. We care about the chemicals used in the process of creating our food, cosmetics and toiletries, clothing, and other goods. We are concerned about whether people were treated unfairly in order to bring it to our tables, bathrooms, closets, and lives, and what animals might have been harmed in the process. We care because we care about ourselves and our primary home, our bodies. But we cannot care about ourselves without caring about our planetary home, Earth. Carl Sagan summarizes it beautifully:

The significance of our lives and our fragile planet is then determined only by our wisdom and courage. We are the custodians of life's meaning. We long for a Parent to care for us, to forgive us our errors, to save us from our childish mistakes. But knowledge is preferable to ignorance. Better by far to embrace the hard truth than a reassuring fable.

YOUR INVITATION TO PRACTICE HEALTH

To care for ourselves and our world then becomes, for each of us, the very definition of what it means to thrive.

1. I invite you to visit health-conscious.org and view link to the pictures collected from various space probes of our Universe. In the mass of stars, gas, asteroids is our tiny, fragile home we call Earth.

2. Can you see yourself standing there beside your glossy Mercedes, talking on your cell phone in the context of these amazing pictures?

202 | **THE 7 PRINCIPLES OF HEALTH**

3. Now ask yourself this question as you stare at this picture: What is really important in the grand scheme of things, as viewed from the big picture? Take a minute to list at least two things which are significant to you.

(1) _____

(2) _____

4. Now, ask yourself this final question: What am I going to do to change my future?

_____

_____

_____

_____

_____

●

"How would you change the world?" I ask Destiny.

She sits on the edge of the green exam table, wearing a black and white checked hat that's slouched over her long, dark locks. She's 16 years old, with a sullen mouth and liquid doe eyes hiding behind thick glasses, not unlike most teenagers these days. Suddenly, she perks up. The corner of her lip curls into a smile as she sits straight, suddenly interested.

Her mother bursts out laughing. "Wow! Now that's a question, isn't it Des?!" she exclaims.

"It's not possible," she replies, her huge eyes the size of headlights. "I can't stand the *muggles*!" She gestures hopelessly with her hand.

"Neither can I," I murmur and ask her to take off her glasses to read the eye chart. "But seriously, you're going to inherit this world. How would you change it?"

PRINCIPLE 7: HEAL, CHANGE, AND THRIVE | 203

Destiny's eyebrows knit together as she sets her mouth into a pout. "I can't," she states flatly, dropping her voice. "Why not?" I persist.

"Because I can't use magic. Now, if I could use magic..."

"But you can," I tell her. "It's just a different type of magic than Harry Potter uses."

"No, I can't!" she protests, staring at me as if I'm crazy.

"Oh, yes, you can," I insist, smiling and handing back her glasses. "Here, put these on. Do you see anything different?" She nods. "Remember, all you have to do is first change yourself in tiny ways — you know, baby steps. It's not so hard. And if you can do that, you *can* change your world!"

CHAPTER TEN

Epilogue

"It's not easy to be a pioneer — but oh, it is fascinating! I would not trade
one moment, even the worst moment, for all the riches in the world."

— **Elizabeth Blackwell, M.D.** *(1821-1910)*
First woman in the United States to earn a medical degree

People tell me stories all the time. It's my job to listen. But there's one
last story I'd like to share with you before we say goodbye. This one is
my story.

●

I've always known there was something more to medicine than just
dishing out prescriptions and telling people what to do for their
health. But my career started in the confines of emergency rooms and
doctors' offices in Canada, busy places to practice medicine. People
came in worried about their problems, not searching for health. I was
trained to focus on disease. I was trained to fix things. I didn't have
time to sit around and chat with Mrs. Richardson while she told me
about the relationship problems that were causing her physical symptoms.

She had the flu. Again. It was the sixth time she'd been in to see
us for an infectious disease, but I really didn't want to hear about the
stress in her life. I didn't have time. Doctors know how that goes —
once we ask someone what's going on in their life, we would never be
able to get out of the exam room. Angry people are waiting outside for
their turn, too. We doctors were too busy to find the real causes of our
patients' problems; we only had time to treat their diseases.

EPILOGUE | 205

Many doctors call it the "hand on the door" sign. Just as we're about to leave the exam room with our hand on the door, the patient says, "Oh, Doctor. There's one more thing. Do you have a second?"

As the years passed, I began to notice in my patients' eyes that there was something more they wanted to say, but the words wouldn't form on their lips. And I knew that if I let them share what was really on their minds, I'd never get through my hectic day. There were so many people with so many things to say. And no one, me included, had the time to listen.

Youth Is Wasted on the Young

I'll admit I was once young and foolish. I'd started practicing medicine by age 25 and I didn't have the experience to talk about things that concerned middle-aged or elderly people. How was I supposed to even pretend to look like I understood their lives? But talk to me about their rash or kidney infection — yeah, I could relate to all that. I could fix their problems.

More years passed. I saw more and more diseases walk in my office door. But I began to see something else. That look in my patients' eyes, just as I was about to leave the room, kept haunting me. I began to recognize it over and over again as it showed up in many different faces, and I knew that it wasn't going to be a short story. I'd been down this road with a few other patients. And whenever I allowed them to tell me their stories, my day would finish hours later, and I'd be ten times more exhausted than if I'd quietly left the room without bothering to ask.

During those years in Canada, I found myself working harder and harder. But soon the government began to blame doctors for the cost of healthcare. They turned a blind eye to the multimillions of dollars paid to hockey players, but they would blame remote-area doctors who worked twenty-six hours a day, eight days a week, expecting them to accept tough love as payment.

So I left the country.

At the ripe old age of 29, after four-and-a-half years in medical practice, I knew that my destiny lay in capitalist America. At least down there in what Canadians called "gun-toting Arizona," they didn't blame

206 | THE 7 PRINCIPLES OF HEALTH

doctors for doing well in their professions, especially since it was such a necessary and noble one. Besides, Bill and Hillary Clinton were desperate for my kind of doctor in the country; cost-effective primary care providers who would be the gatekeepers of healthcare. They made it easy for me to get a job and a green card.

A few years later, it turned out that Bill and Hillary Clinton didn't get what they wanted. Nor did the rest of America. It's just that we both didn't know it at the time.

Glory Days

The years from 2000 to about 2003 were what I call my glory years. I became specialized in acute care medicine, a field now known as urgent care, a growing one for primary care doctors like me. I was employed with a large hospital system where I worked hard and received decent pay. But as I continued to focus more on disease care and acute problems, my patients' eyes continued to haunt me. Something was wrong. More and more of them had that same look, but I couldn't put my finger on it. I had this growing sense of paralysis inside me that was spreading like a cancer, yet I couldn't identify the feeling, because I loved what I did and thought I was making a difference in my patients' lives. So I just kept going, writing more prescriptions and shoving my patients gently out the door, moving on to the next person who needed help.

Suddenly, in 2003, my glorious world fell apart. The large hospital system announced that it was going to shut down all the urgent care clinics I had helped to grow. Inside of one month, I'd be out of a job. Worse, there was nowhere else I wanted to go. I loved the staff I worked with; they had become family. We had done well for many, many people and had truly helped them. I didn't want to move on, but reality was knocking at my door, so I decided that instead of working for someone else, I'd make a go of setting up my own clinic.

Dreams

I had a vision, a dream. I wanted to see if I could help my patients in a different way and somehow stop their haunted looks. But I also knew that I couldn't do it all myself. I was the disease doctor and I enjoyed

EPILOGUE | 207

what I did in that role. It was my niche, and I did it well. But I knew my patients would benefit if I could do what I did best, and then show them another way to find real health — with someone who actually practiced health.

So I teamed up with my younger sister. She'd studied to be a chiropractor, and was constantly challenged by the fact she'd grown up in our family of conventional medical doctors. Dad would tease her about being a quack, lovingly of course. He was the ultimate paternalistic medical doctor. We all joked about her "heebie-jeebie" practices. As conventionally trained practitioners, we knew we were the *real* doctors. There was a certain truth to Dad's jokes — or so we all believed.

My sister didn't seem to be bothered. She kept telling us that we needed to watch what we ate, be aware of all the chemicals in our water, and take plenty of fish-oil supplements. She told us that acupuncture would help us heal. She told us to get massages every week for therapeutic purposes.

We all laughed at her.

But by 2005, the sound of my laugh wasn't quite so loud. When I wrote my business plan for the new clinic, my research showed that patients were paying cash out of their pockets for complementary and alternative medicine. I figured out that we could set up an urgent care clinic mixed with a chiropractic office in the same building, something that was very unusual at the time. On the urgent care side of the clinic, we would likely see patients only once for their problems. But on the chiropractic side, we would be able to treat them over several visits and really help them back to optimal health.

Could this be what patients need? I wondered. *Could this be the type of healthcare service I was looking to offer my patients that would stop the mounting worry and stress I detected in their eyes every day?*

I began to struggle to put together this business model, but health insurance companies would have none of it. They didn't understand what a chiropractor was doing in an urgent care clinic. They made it very difficult to get our unique clinic contracted as part of their so-called "healthcare provider network." Patients didn't understand the concept either. "I just want a pill for my pain," they would say. Doctors didn't understand. "What's a chiropractor doing in urgent care clinic?" they would ask sarcastically. "Crack 'em and whack 'em, ey?" They thought *I* was a quack — a loving and loveable lunatic.

And then reality came knocking, again. This time it broke down the door.

During that first year, as we paid thousands of dollars a month in rent, the lady who was supposed to be doing our medical billing had decided not do her job — for *four months.* I trusted her, as she had worked with me at the large hospital company before. Now I realized that they had been the lucky ones.

Then, the large corporation from which we rented our strip mall office had their anchor grocery store tenant default on opening for 18 months. We and a handful of other small businesses limped along for more than a year without the higher volume foot traffic which would have been attracted by a grocery store anchor. The health insurance companies took their own sweet time with allowing our contracts to get in-network on their provider lists. They acted as though they were doing *us* a favor, while *their* patients were denied access to healthcare services, and we were denied participating in their networks. Patients would walk out of the office in a huff, wondering what was wrong with us. They had no interest in listening to the reality that doctors had to live through in setting up their own practices and trying to get contracted with these corporate giants who controlled everything to do with healthcare delivery.

Then, after living on loans for months until we could get paid, our largest health insurance company payer, whose money we so desperately needed to keep the lights on, breeched our signed contract with them. Their several billion dollar computer system decided to kick all our claims to out-of-network status. That meant that hundreds of thousands of dollars in payments we were due got mailed directly to our patients for services that we had provided. It was as if a grocery store's third-party distributor was paying its customers to shop and consume their products, instead of it being the other way around!

Was this just the way capitalist America worked? I wondered. *Or was this capitalist healthcare run amok, where we weren't the ones allowed to be capitalists, but Wall Street was?*

When we asked the health insurance company to fix the problems they had caused, they kept us — entangled in administrative

EPILOGUE | 209

red-tape for months while our bank account drained. Finally, as I mentioned in an earlier chapter, I got in my car, drove to their headquarters, and demanded to see their CEO. I was prepared to sit in their lobby and get arrested if I had to. I was going to call all the news channels. What they had done was so unfair to us as the little guy struggling to make a living by just being a good doctor.

A year later, America's healthcare crisis blossomed on the media horizon, and another large health insurance company decided to delay our contracts, forcing our patients to seek care in more expensive emergency rooms. The insurance behemoth didn't care. It was just the way they did things, they said. "Contracts take a long time, Doctor — deal with it."

Their inaction was crippling our fledgling company. My life savings hemorrhaged, year after year, as I wondered why I had chosen medicine as a career. Nobody seemed to care about the huge struggles we faced as doctors trying to operate a small business. I wondered what kind of career a high school graduate would choose if they were told they would be forced to pay everyone else in order to stay in business as part of their profession. I wondered if America really understood the consequences of shooting quality doctors in the chest in this way. I'd lived through the Canadian healthcare system and moved on; yet suddenly, only a few years later, Canada was once again making it enticing to stay in my profession because they had quickly realized that without doctors, the single-payer government could not actually provide healthcare to its people.

Nightmares

I knew I wasn't alone. My colleagues were increasingly disillusioned. They were struggling with health insurance companies like thousands of tiny "Davids" up against a handful of merciless Goliaths. They were working longer and harder, and getting burned out in their mid-30s. I could hear it in their voices, just a few years after graduation. Their enthusiasm for life and for making a difference in the world by helping others, a noble profession in any other context, soon gave way to exhaustion and bitterness. I knew they were facing hundreds of thousands of dollars in student loans they could never pay off in their

210 | THE 7 PRINCIPLES OF HEALTH

lifetimes. Instead of trust funds, their kids would inherit debt. So they told their kids to do anything other than go into medicine as a career.

Like every great type A woman who ever lived, I began to work harder, believing it was me who somehow wasn't doing enough. So I ran around faster. I multitasked my way to multitasking. I knew the services we offered, the integrated skills of disease and wellness, were what patients truly needed, but the world wasn't listening. Patients were consumed with their disease mindsets, and the problem grew worse every year. The haunted look that first began showing up in my patients' eyes was now manifesting as physical diseases in their bodies. Everyone everywhere was getting sicker: mentally, physically, and emotionally. And now, financial illness was settling in, too.

I did what I was trained to do. I kept dishing out medications, thinking it would help. I kept recommending that my patients visit my sister, the chiropractic doctor, for healthcare if they wanted to get well.

"Are her services covered by insurance?" they would ask.

"No, but you'll spend much, much less in the long run if you take care of yourself now," I responded rationally.

No one seemed to understand, least of all the patients. Deductibles continued to skyrocket. Coverage for real wellness care dropped. People got sicker and sicker. And still, patients would ask, "Are her services covered by insurance?" People didn't seem to understand that if they just did the calculations, they would see that they'd spent infinitely less on wellness care than they would for the bureaucracy of health insurance that drastically limited true healthcare.

I kept going, stuck now in this fight for my life and my career. I was heavily invested in our clinics, and I really believed in them. I believed in my sister and the care she provided. She had helped me avoid a surgery that my own gynecologist had recommended. She was able to keep me from needing prescription pills. She was a true, gifted healer.

Then the financial crash of 2008 happened, and we all reeled from the impact.

Then my father died. I collapsed from that hit, but eventually I got back up on weak legs.

Then our new billing company suddenly dropped us as a client

EPILOGUE | 211

— out of spite — a month after my father died. This was the third billing company we had used, in fact, but it was also a small mom-and-pop outfit. The owner got wind that I knew she wasn't doing her job. We were making a business move to switch billing companies again, so she decided to upend us before we could fire her, the day after I flew home to my father's funeral in Canada.

Then Medicare decided to audit our clinics. Just because.

Then I was served with a subpoena for a large malpractice suit that involved multiple parties.

Then the same large health insurance company I mentioned before breeched our contract *again*, for *exactly* the same reason they had a few years earlier. They claimed it was a glitch in their multibillion dollar computer system. Again, just because.

Then the government decided to hold back more payments to all doctors nationwide, because of the increasing debt loads on the Medicare program.

Then, health insurance companies began to cut back more and more in payments to doctors under their classic excuse, "It costs more for healthcare these days." All despite posting double-digit profit margins for their stockholders during the worst years of America's recession.

Somehow, I made it to 2009, when I was diagnosed with high blood pressure.

Then I was diagnosed with early diabetes.

Then my thyroid gland decided to weaken, along with my adrenal glands, ovaries, cholesterol, vitamin D, and lower back.

Then I said to the Universe, "I freaking quit!! *You* figure this out!"

What's Going to Kill Me First?

My genetics were catching up with me, but I couldn't afford to care for myself. I worked like crazy. I was stressed out. I was living in the hell that is called healthcare in America today, but would better be called *hell*-care. That's when my body took control and decided to shut down. My mind was shutting down at the same time. My finances were shutting down. My life was slipping away, in front of my eyes. I never would have believed that before the age of 45, I would feel like an 80-year-old.

212 | THE 7 PRINCIPLES OF HEALTH

In September 2010, my entire body system suddenly began to reject all food. I had been working hard, as usual, going weeks without a break, when I began getting ill with fever and chills. I felt exhausted every day, despite sleeping for eight hours most nights. I knew my immune system was stressed. One thing about our Dad: he was old school and allowed our bodies to fight infection naturally when we were kids, despite his paternalistic attitude. That gave us the immunity of 10,000 horses.

But, when I became sick, I knew my immune system was very weak. When my body began to reject all the foods I liked — meat, cheese, bread, pasta, rice — I couldn't understand what was going on, even though I was a doctor! It was so very strange. I finally put it down to some sort of virus that wouldn't allow me to eat but still allowed me to work. Every time I tried to put a morsel of food into my mouth, I suddenly felt nauseated. Meat: instantly rejected. Dairy: not happening. Fast food: are you kidding? Eggs, my favorite, smelled like dead animal to me. I couldn't eat a thing — for a whole month. I don't know how I lived, but I did, on about 600 calories a day. No exaggeration. My fat stores must have been enough to keep me alive.

I lost weight, to the tune of 30 pounds, and began to think I might have a tumor. But I also began to feel better. Could I have a cancer that was making me feel great? My sister laughed at me. It was her turn to get me back on track.

I was too depleted, energetically, to continue my heavy weight-lifting and running workouts, so I stopped them entirely. I stopped whipping myself for not meeting my personal bests in every activity I endeavored. I decided to take up the practice of yoga, but avoided going to any classes where I would compare myself to the lady on the mat next to me. I stopped thinking that I was not good enough for not being good enough. I bought one of Rodney Yee's yoga books, and resolved to practice yoga every day, exactly as he advised, no matter how I was feeling. I resolved to show up every day to my mat and do only what I could, without judging myself.

Slowly, as I stayed on my mat, things began to change. I wasn't eating well during this time, but I was still practicing medicine and running my company. Slowly, as I came back to my mat every day in the silence and the darkness of my life, I began to crave this time more

EPILOGUE | 213

than I did food. I needed the quiet space. I cherished it. Suddenly, the noise that had surrounded me all my life decreased in volume, and I found myself in the most amazing place.

40 Days and 40 Nights

It took about 40 days. I practiced a little bit every day, showing up on my mat, crying on it, loving it, moving my body, experiencing the world around me, and opened my mind to space. I continued to change. As I kept at it, I began to understand something profound. I began to understand the meaning of Principle 1, *Be Present*.

I can't tell you what it was like to eat real food again after 40 days. Everything tasted incredible! I hadn't been a big vegetable eater, but now veggies tasted like ambrosia. My lips couldn't touch any type of meat, except seafood. It was as though my brain had reprogrammed its thoughts to being a fanatical vegetarian. I began to prepare vegetarian meals, and enjoyed every bite as though it were my last. I didn't regret a thing about my sudden diet change, although I'd yo-yo dieted along with the best of them. I began to appreciate every moment of my life through my experience of now being able to eat, smell, and taste to full capacity once again. I began to *live*.

This is the point when I began to understand Principle 2, *Become Aware*.

Suddenly, I was aware of myself. I was looking great — fantastic, in fact. I was approaching my mid-40s, and I was feeling the best I'd ever felt in my life. I was lifting more weight than I'd ever lifted before in my workouts, despite having goal after goal with my personal trainer. I was standing on my head and twisting my body into strange shapes; I was doing things I had never done as a kid!

Thoughts about the stresses of work began to drift away during these precious moments. My worries about healthcare and the future of the world receded. It's not that things magically improved. It's just that somehow things kept going for us at the clinics. What happened instead was that I began to recognize my own thought patterns in the silence I had created every day. I saw that ruminating about past events or worrying about a future I couldn't control was taking me away from my experience of this world right now. I became very

THE 7 PRINCIPLES OF HEALTH

aware of how much time I was wasting in those moments, so I began to make different choices to feed my mind, just as I had made different choices to feed my body.

My mind began to enjoy a new diet of healthful thoughts! I became aware of a few things about healthcare, many of which I've outlined in this book. I became aware of my role as a doctor and as a human being, and aware of my past attempts to struggle through it all. I became, almost suddenly, aware of what I had to do next.

This is when I decided how I was going to live. I was not going to live in disease, like my colleagues and I had been trained to do for our patients. I was going to live every moment of every day in health and happiness, first. I finally understood the meaning of Principle 3, *Be Health*.

The Rest Is History

Once I arrived at this point, there was no stopping me! I now understood Principle 4, *Reawaken Curiosity*. I had already been gifted with that principle through my sister. Though I'd once laughed at her, I now realized that she had been trained in the health paradigm we all had to find someday.

So yes, I became a quack-lover! And a massage therapist-lover! And a hypnotherapist-lover. And a Chinese Medicine doctor-lover. And an herbalogist-lover. And a lover of the many, many other wonderful health practitioners I've met along my journey and have yet to meet; practitioners who have shown and will continue to show me how terribly wrong we've been in conventional medicine all this time. My thoughts were so misguided all those years ago. I now see the light and the darkness inside which we live in healthcare and in America.

I've stopped listening to the programmed messages and toxic noise of an out-dated medical system. I've opened my eyes and shifted my thoughts to understand a very different paradigm. I've awakened from my nightmare and become conscious.

And wow! What an amazing world I see!

Principle 5, *Channel Creativity*, is a concept I created to teach you how I developed my own health network. As you've learned, this is called a health-centric model and will one day become widely accepted as the standard healthcare model from which we must operate if we are to find our way to optimal health. The health providers and practitioners in my network are the most amazing people who I know will guide me to feel more youthful and energetic for a long time to come. And I share all of them with you on my website.

Principle 6, *Grow and Renew*, reminds us of what and who we are. For some reason, we've forgotten this natural law along the way in medicine. And we've all forgotten who we are. It's time to be and live our truth and our connection to each other and this world instead of disguising it through modern healthcare.

Principle 7, *Heal, Change, and Thrive*, is manifested in this book. I know I have healed, from the outside-in, and the inside-out. I love that I have changed. I'm positive that I will thrive.

One question, however, still remains. Will *you* choose to do it, too?

The Power to Heal

Only you can determine your power to heal, not some outside party with its own financial or political agenda. Decide in this moment how you will live before you die. Release the fear, distraction, and disempowerment which infuse our society and today's medical system and resolve to no longer live as a victim. Resolve to change yourself. Journey with me as we reinvent health through the *Health Conscious Movement.*

And then, resolve to change your world.

Yours in health consciousness,
natasha
Chandler, Arizona
March 2013

ACKNOWLEDGMENTS

In producing such a book that comes directly from the heart, it's often difficult to know whom to thank first. So many have contributed to my education and enlightenment, both formal and informal, along this journey we call life. I'll give my best shot here, yet remain in the uncomfortable realization that these words couldn't even begin to convey the level of gratitude I feel as I write them.

First, to every one of my patients who have taught me, beginning at the tender young age of 25, to quell my arrogance and fear, introspect at the deepest levels about who I am and what I'm doing here, and emerge with a conviction so strong, I am now willing to do everything it takes to undo the wrongs that our healthcare industry has inflicted on all of us. Thanks is not enough for the ways you have shaped my thoughts by unselfishly offering me glimpses into those sacred parts of your lives. May we each find our way to freedom from the health-fear we've created and served to you as the healthcare system we understand today.

Second, to my incredible husband, who stood by my side through thick and thicker, holding out his hand patiently for me to clutch every time I stumbled. Roger, you are truly my best friend, my rock, and my sunshine and I love you to the far reaches of the Universe and back! QT3.1415.

To those who took my crazy idea and helped shape it into what you hold in your hands and what you experience through our social media outlets. Bob "Merlin" Davis who, when I first met him, believed beyond a shadow of a doubt in my magic. To "The Girls": Kerrisa Olson, Maria Chavez, and Mary Zook who stood by me, confident that one day I would do it, while you watched my self-torture in trying to perfect this message. To my brother, Dr. Dinesh Deonarain, who put me up

218 | ACKNOWLEGMENTS

in tiny New Zealand hotel rooms staring into green country pastures as I wrote the first draft of this book; you are truly Apollo to my Diana! And to my sister, Dr. Sharena Deonarain, who was right all along.

To Brian Nowak who, when he heard my visions, told his Facebook community, "This is epic!" To my best friend Mary K. and her personal fight that's opened my eyes to the meaning of our lives together. To all my staff, business partners, colleagues and associates along the way who have been witness to my personal and professional changes over the years. Daryn Krywko, thank you for believing in me with one business and helping me transition safely to another.

To each of my reviewers: Dr. Gladys McGarey, Dr. Larry Malerba, Naomi Rhode, Don Thoren, and Steve Cadwell. You are all truly amazing, and I am honored to be a part of shaping a new future together with you.

To Laura Orsini, my editor; you have navigated these waters expertly along the way to this book's fruition. You've led me to those who most count and whom I can most count on: Sam Sites, Bill Greaves, and Scott White – our journey together has just begun! I can't wait for the next chapter!

To my mother, Mary Shiela Penelope Deonarain. As dad used to say, "You are only a teacher. But you've stood patiently inside our family of stubborn doctors until we finally learned how to listen."

And last but certainly not least — for you would never allow that — to my father, Dr. Pramjee Deonarain. Dad, a day hasn't gone by when I haven't thought about you since you died. And now I understand why you taught me the way you did. I am proud to say I've learned my lesson; you've taught me well. And I'm proud to know that I am your daughter, not just in flesh, but in spirit too. May I truly be as strong in my convictions and as fearless as you were, all the days of my life.

ABOUT THE AUTHOR

Natasha N. Deonarain, MD, MBA

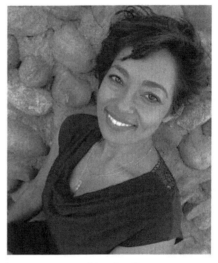

With 20+ years as a conventionally trained physician who has owned and operated cutting-edge, integrated medical clinics, Dr. Natasha Deonarain brings her leadership and entrepreneurial experience to fruition in this undertaking to transform the delivery of healthcare.

In *The 7 Principles of Health*, she discusses how external stakeholders have united in their strong drive for profit, heavily influencing doctors to operate from a disease-focused perspective, thus leading us to paradoxically create more disease under the guise of healthcare.

As a solution to this paradox, Dr. Deonarain has founded the **Health Conscious Movement**, which uses multiple social media channels to deliver a call to health consciousness. Its mission is to bring doctors, patients, organizations, institutions, communities — and YOU — together as one, in a massive collaborative learning experience that will transform the delivery of healthcare by implementing this exciting new paradigm.

INDEX

#

5 Components of Total Health 44-45, 102, 164, 172-174, 176, 183-184, 186

5 Disciplines of Health Practice 12, 36, 37, 41, 49, 112, 133, 183

7 Habits of Highly Effective People 9

7 Principles of Health 10, 11, 27-30, 32, 36, 49, 50, 51, 52, 112, 130, 133, 178, 182, 183, 197, 198, 200

    PRINCIPLE 1: Be Present 30-31

    PRINCIPLE 2: Become Aware 31-32

    PRINCIPLE 3: Be Health 33

    PRINCIPLE 4: Reawaken Curiosity 33-34

    PRINCIPLE 5: Channel Creativity 34-35

    PRINCIPLE 6: Grow and Renew 35

    PRINCIPLE 7: Heal, Change, and Thrive 35-36

7 Requirements for Health Practice 12, 46, 49, 125, 183

    Commitment 46, 49, 125

    Desire 46, 49, 125

    Lifelong View 46, 49, 125

    Outside-in, Inside-out 125

    Self-Accountability 125

    Sequential Steps 125

    Small Steps 125

19-year-old man's story 58-59

A

absence of disease 26, 62-63, 73, 102, 117, 131, 169

Accepting 36-37, 40, 112
    See also 5 Disciplines of Health Practice

accountability: *See* Self-Accountability

action vs. reaction 133

acupuncture 23, 67, 101, 107-108, 124, 135-136, 146, 152-155, 182-183, 188, 207

AED: *See* automated external defibrilator

Agus, Dr. David 184

Allison's story 23-25, 27, 102, 160

Armstrong, Lance 101

art 108, 146

astrology
    as healing modality 108

astronomy 18, 51

automated external defibrillator 54, 191

awareness 13, 15, 91, 92, 99
    consciousness and 13

B

balance 10, 30-31, 35, 44-45, 58, 76,

81, 102, 144, 147, 173, 174, 179, 189
definition 15
health 30
law of 30
life and 30

baseline
creating a new 184-186

Become Aware 31-32, 40, 71-72, 103, 116, 129-133, 150-151, 178, 213
five senses 31-32

behavior 55, 61, 99, 140, 149, 172
modification 55, 61

Be Health 33, 40, 98-102, 105, 108, 110-111, 116-118, 130, 151, 152, 178, 184, 214
vs. become healthy 33

belief systems 23, 50-52, 93, 105, 110, 121, 137

Be Present 30, 31, 40, 53, 56, 69, 70, 72, 103, 128, 130, 131, 132, 133, 150, 178, 196, 213

Bertillion, Jacques 20

big picture perspective 13, 18, 22, 27, 29, 51, 60, 73, 76, 89, 91, 140, 141, 173, 202
astronomy and 51
healthcare and 18, 22, 27, 29, 60, 73, 76, 89, 140, 173
paradigm shift 18
view from outer space 51

Blackwell, Dr. Elizabeth 204

blame 4, 23, 48, 70, 76, 81-83, 111, 127, 140, 205

Bloomberg Businessweek 75

Blue Cross and Blue Shield 77

body image 100

Bossier de Lacroix, François 20

brain-mapping 99

Brantley, Timothy 94, 173

Brittney's story 94-95

Buddha: *See* Siddhartha Gautama

C

CAM: *See* Complimentary and Alternative Medicine

cancer 23, 27, 33, 34, 39-40, 43, 55, 60, 62, 64-65, 80, 94, 101-105, 122, 139, 141, 160, 173, 206, 212
asparagus as treatment 55, 60, 139
cost 74
lemons as treatment 55, 60

Candy's story 84

Catherine's story 138-145

chakra healers 108

change 3, 5, 9, 12, 18, 19, 24-25, 26-28, 28-30, 37, 47-52, 55-60, 68, 76, 93, 94, 96, 100, 102, 103, 109, 115, 124, 125, 127-130, 132-134, 136, 139, 141, 151, 155, 160, 161, 164, 174, 179-181, 186, 189, 194-196, 198, 202-203, 212-213, 215
individuals and 12
physical 76, 100
requirements for 26
society and 27

Channel Creativity 34, 40, 143, 145, 149, 154, 179, 214

checkup 8, 21, 35, 131, 166-169, 180, 183
as a screen for disease 8

paradoxical practice 8

Chinese Medicine 23, 107, 117, 214

Chopra M.D., Deepak 53, 152

clairvoyants 108, 183

Clark, Jim 99

clear vision 15, 92, 142, 193
   definition 15

clinical evidence 107

Clinton, Bill and Hillary 206

collaboration 15, 92, 124

collective 5, 9, 12, 14, 23-24, 90, 91, 93, 197.
   See also whole
   ability to find health 5
   definition 14
   mindset 23
   vs. individual interests 90

Commitment 46, 47-48, 128.
   See also 7 Requirements for Health Practice

common sense 20, 61, 131, 134, 155

Complementary and Alternative Medicine 56, 87, 181, 182, 207

conscious 11, 13, 25, 49, 52, 70, 81, 91, 112, 144, 161, 162, 201, 214
   vs. subconscious 110
   vs. unconscious 13

consciousness
   and health 11
   definition 15

consumers 75, 181-182
   as patients 181

Cooper, Hillary 28

Copernicus 17

Cosby, Bill 127

Covey, Stephen 9, 12, 19, 124

creation 10, 22, 143, 164, 172, 179, 182
   create first in thought 7-10
   in healthcare 143, 182
   manifest thoughts in physical form 19
   thoughts and thought forms 19-23

creativity 34, 40, 143, 145-149, 154-155, 179, 214
   and innate ability to heal 40
   left-brain thinking 146
   right-brain thinking 146

cure 13, 16-17, 21-22, 35, 40, 47, 48, 61, 67, 83, 90, 100, 105, 120, 122, 123, 136, 141, 153, 193
   vs. heal 142, 193

curiosity 33, 40, 122, 124, 130, 138-143, 153, 178, 214
   and desperation 141
   and distraction 138-140
   and innate ability to heal 40

Current Health Paradigm 12, 15, 61, 65, 89, 90, 94, 95, 101, 102, 106, 133, 134, 141, 142, 160, 182, 192, 193

cycles 164

D

David's story 62, 63

Da Vinci, Leonardo 37

defensive medicine 82-83, 122
   costs 83

degenerative diseases 80, 129

de Lacroix, François Bossier 20

Desire 46-48, 126, 128.
   See also 7 Requirements for Health
   Practice

Destiny's story 202-203

diabetes 63, 74, 86, 88, 103-105, 130, 138-140, 160, 170, 211
   cost 74

dis-ease 14, 41, 92, 117, 150

disease 5, 8, 12, 14, 16-18, 20-25, 26-27, 32, 34-35, 38, 41, 43, 44, 48, 50, 52, 55, 61, 62-68, 73-77, 78-80, 81, 85, 86, 88, 92, 93-94, 95-96, 99-105, 106, 107, 112, 114, 117, 118, 120-123, 126-127, 129-133, 136, 139-141, 143, 144, 147, 148-150, 151, 152, 153, 155, 156, 157, 160-161, 166, 167, 168-169, 170, 172-175, 176-178, 179, 180-183, 184-188, 193, 195-196, 204, 206, 207, 210, 214.
   See also disease-focused thinking
   as a challenge 38, 40, 51, 100, 104, 195
   as currency 50, 89, 93
   as empowerment 43
   as opportunity 41-43
   labeling 22, 26-27, 33, 35, 43-44, 52, 63, 88, 102-105, 148, 152-153, 187

disease currency: *See* disease, as currency

disease, death, and dying 61, 77
   as a thought system 8
   focus on 8

disease-fix-cure paradigm 67

disease-focused medical system 22, 34, 50, 63, 76, 80, 105, 149, 167-168, 176, 179, 181, 183, 186, 195

disease-focused thinking 5, 8, 20, 22, 23, 34-35, 41, 50, 63, 67, 73, 76, 80, 88, 105, 106, 122, 132, 139-143, 149, 151, 167-168, 175, 176, 178, 179, 181, 183, 186, 193, 195

disease labels 88, 103-105, 148, 152-153, 187
   doctors and 103, 152

disease network 120, 143-144

disease orientation
   definition 90

disease-oriented: *See* disease-focused thinking

disease paradigm 25

Disease Triangle 42

disempowerment 13, 60-63, 65, 70, 76, 83, 88, 90, 94, 103, 116, 128, 142, 179, 194, 215

Disney, Walt 189

distraction 5, 30, 60-65, 76, 89, 103, 111, 116, 125, 128, 132, 138-142, 178, 194, 215

divorce 128

docēre 87

doctor-patient relationship 4, 22-23, 38, 56, 76, 82-83, 87-88

doctors 2, 4-5, 7-9, 11, 12, 14-16, 20-25, 25-30, 26, 27, 32, 33, 34, 37, 40, 43-44, 47, 52, 54, 56, 57, 61, 62, 63, 64-65, 66, 68, 73, 78-79, 82-83, 85, 86-90, 99, 101-104, 106-109, 110, 112, 120, 122-124, 126-127, 128, 129, 130, 136, 139, 143, 148, 149, 150-151, 152, 154-157, 161, 166, 168-169, 170, 175, 178, 180-185, 193, 198, 204-211, 217
   and acupuncture 23, 107

THE 7 PRINCIPLES OF HEALTH

and alternative medicine 23

and blame 127

and Chinese Medicine 23, 107

and chiropractic 23

and Eastern medicine 23

and fear 122

and homeopathy 153

and naturopathy 23

as authority figures 87

as guides 15, 142

as healers 52

as healthcare stakeholders 87-89

conventionally trained 8, 22, 34, 38, 65, 75, 88, 107-109, 123-124, 146-147, 149-150, 152, 155, 157, 182, 185, 207

dictates 13, 49, 91, 108, 144, 175

dogma 51-52, 107, 162

education 51, 122-123

ego and judgment 52, 106-109, 144, 183

orders 13, 40, 49, 82, 87, 91

parent/child relationship 13, 87, 91

paternalism 13, 91, 94

programming disease 27

questioning their authority 87

specialists 3, 62, 88-89, 123, 140, 148, 150-151, 172, 186

training 51-52, 63, 73, 85, 112, 123, 139, 161

dogma 51-52, 107, 162

Donne, John 199

Don's story 67-68, 160, 191, 193

Dr. Duncan's story 67

Dr. Oz 139, 140

Dr. Seuss 119, 144

drug companies 8, 25, 73, 83-85, 102
as healthcare stakeholders 83-85

drug resistance 66-67, 84

Dyer, Dr. Wayne 145, 152

E

Earth 16-18, 136, 198, 201
changing perspectives 16
Copernicus and the Sun 17
geocentric belief vs. heliocentric belief 16-17

Eastern medicine 13, 23, 90, 123, 146, 187

ego 31, 52, 86, 103, 106-109, 112, 123, 136, 144, 155, 157, 175, 178, 183, 194
and judgment 52, 112, 123, 175, 178-179, 183, 194

Einstein, Albert 5, 14, 17, 123, 194

Eliot, George 192

emergency rooms 66, 82-83, 113-116, 204, 209

emotional stress 76

empowerment 15-16, 43, 61, 89, 92, 103, 131-133, 142, 155, 160, 178, 183, 187
definition 15
in healthcare choices 16, 92, 131, 160, 183

energetic system
definition 14

energy 14, 17, 19, 47, 92, 107-108, 117-118, 137, 149-150, 153, 176, 183, 185, 187-188, 195
prana 117

qi 117-118, 185

energy healing 47, 108, 137, 183, 188

energy medicine: *See* energy healing

energy practitioner: *See* energy healing

epidemics 16, 34, 79, 103, 160
  paradoxical creation of 16, 45

excuses 39, 48, 70

external stakeholders: *See* healthcare stakeholders

F

Favre, Brett 161

FDA 85, 152

fear 5, 20, 22, 32, 36-42, 44, 45, 63-66, 68, 73, 76-77, 80-81, 88-89, 94, 103-104, 108-112, 110, 116-118, 122, 122-125, 127-128, 130, 133-134, 139, 141-142, 155, 157, 178-179, 182, 185-186, 194-197, 215, 216
  and health insurance profits 80
  of death 44, 64, 81, 133, 141
  fear vs. curiosity 122

finding health 5, 18, 19, 23, 26, 30-31, 37, 39, 41, 43-44, 45, 47, 50-51, 57-58, 65, 70, 72, 89, 102-103, 106, 109, 110, 112, 123, 125, 127, 133-136, 138-143, 150-151, 160, 186
  balance and 31, 45
  by focusing on disease 5, 26

Flipbook Medical Exam 168

Ford, Henry 108

fragmentation 12, 90
  definition 90

Franklin, Benjamin 129

Frank's story 141-142

G

Gandhi, Mahatma 57, 133

gap 45, 52, 59, 61, 72, 83, 104, 143, 178, 192
  being in the 59, 143
  moment of silence 56-57
  Stimulus, Gap, Action 143

Gerber M.D., Richard 180, 185-186

global community 18, 200

goals 19, 28, 48, 50, 128, 132
  health goals 48, 132

government 8, 20, 48, 59, 73, 85-87, 97, 120, 126, 130, 154, 160, 178, 180, 196, 205, 209, 211
  as a healthcare stakeholder 85

Great Recession of 2008 75

greed 45, 52, 81, 129, 133, 198

Grow and Renew 35, 40, 163, 179, 215
  law of growth and renewal 35

guide 15, 92, 142, 180, 185, 193
  definition 15

H

habits 10-11, 25, 26, 28, 34, 35, 41, 50, 102, 129, 138-140, 181, 195
  and practices 11
  as destroyers of health 11, 129
  that promote health 11, 25, 34, 35, 41, 50

"hand on the door" sign. 205

Hashimoto's thyroiditis 187

Heal, Change, and Thrive 35, 40, 190, 192, 197, 215

healer
intuitive 153–154

healing 4, 14, 16, 34, 38, 40, 47, 49, 50–51, 58, 66, 83, 84, 106–109, 111, 112, 117–118, 136–137, 154–155, 157, 173, 180, 183, 185, 188, 193, 198, 200
definition 14
innate source 49, 198

health
and creativity 34, 143
definition 26
health balance 173

healthcare crisis 4, 16, 78, 80, 83, 209

healthcare model 16, 144, 167, 215
new 144

healthcare stakeholders 9, 32, 73, 77–89, 124, 127, 133, 143, 179–181, 185
doctors 87–89
drug companies 83–85
government 85–87
health insurance companies 77–81
lawyers 81–83
profit motives 4, 9, 124, 127, 129, 160
role in driving up costs 77–89

healthcare system 4–5, 7–8, 11, 14, 16, 18, 20–23, 25, 32, 37, 43, 47, 51, 52, 61, 63, 73–76, 78, 90, 99, 101, 103, 109, 118, 122, 126–127, 132, 134, 143, 154, 157, 161, 166–167, 186, 196, 198, 209, 216.
See also medical system

beliefs about 8, 47, 131–132

Canada 209

checkup 131, 166

collective mindset 47, 118, 127, 198

disease focus 22, 51, 61, 63

disease labels 43

foundation of fear 37, 122

future 134, 196

negative messaging 101, 103

profit motives 52, 78, 143

vs. health-fear 37

Health-Centric Model 144, 215
definition 144

health checkup: See checkup

Health Conscious Movement 25, 26, 144, 215, 218

health-conscious.org 70, 81, 112, 144, 161, 162, 201

health-fear 37, 103, 216

health goals 48, 132

health guides 20, 155, 160

health insurance 8, 12, 21–22, 24, 25, 39, 48, 59, 66, 73, 75, 77–81, 82, 86–87, 96, 97, 101, 120, 122, 126–127, 130, 140, 143, 148, 150, 151, 154, 155, 158, 159, 160, 178, 191, 195–196, 207–211
companies 8, 21, 25, 48, 73, 75, 77–81, 101, 120, 126, 143, 154, 207–211
as healthcare stakeholders 207–211

health insurance premiums 22, 75, 78–79
employee contributions 75

228 | THE 7 PRINCIPLES OF HEALTH

Health Integration Manager 160-161, 182, 187

Health Maintenance Organization Act of 1973 77

health network 34-35, 120, 143-144, 147, 155-158, 160-161, 179, 181-183, 186, 214

    vs. disease network 143

health provider 34, 72, 173

health statistics 9, 45, 61, 74-75, 75, 76, 178

Health Triangle 42

herbology 23, 38, 147, 183, 187, 214

high cholesterol 74, 86, 88, 117, 126

    cost 74

H.I.M.: *See* Health Integration Manager

Hippocrates 26

holistic practitioners 153-154

Hope's story 1-3, 4, 7, 186-189

human body 13, 88, 90, 123, 133, 149

Huxley, Aldous 124

Hydrocodone 147

hypertension 62, 74, 86, 95-96, 103, 172

    cost 74

hypnotheraphy 183, 214

I

ICD: *See* International Classification of Diseases

immune system 84, 212

individualism 12, 90

    definition 12

individuals 5, 9, 12, 14, 18, 24, 34, 51-52, 58, 60, 61, 63, 67, 90-91, 93, 134, 155, 179-180, 194, 200

    and collective society 5, 9, 18, 93, 200

    and personal choice 61

    as patients 67

    belief systems 93

    creativity 34

    doctors as 63

    inside the medical system 24

innate ability to heal 10, 34, 40, 50, 58, 61

    reawaken your 10

insanity 149, 183

    definition 149

integration 13, 14, 16-18, 35, 76, 89, 90-92, 93, 123, 144, 149, 169, 172, 174, 179, 183, 184, 185, 186, 187, 210

    as humans 149, 169, 172, 174, 184

    effect on the whole 187

    integrated health 35, 76, 123, 179, 183, 186

    mindset of 144

    with the world 17

intentions 19-20.

    See also goals

International Classification of Diseases 20, 38

intuition 146, 185

intuitive healer 108, 153-155, 185

J

James, William 70

Jeff's story 156-163

Jerry's story 105-106

Jesus Christ 57

Jobs, Steve 149

journey of life 194, 216

journey to health 9, 32-34, 56, 61, 69, 73, 76, 118, 131-133, 142-144, 158, 160, 162, 179

judgment 39, 42, 70, 106-109, 112, 123, 131, 137, 175, 178-180, 183, 194
   and disempowerment 70
   and ego 106-108, 112, 123, 175, 178-180, 183, 194
   and fear 42, 178-180

K

Keller, Helen 57

Kellogg M.D., John Harvey 98

King Jr., Martin Luther 50, 57

Kiyosaki, Robert 143

Krishnamurti, Jiddu 134

Kübler-Ross, Elizabeth 163

L

laws 10, 35, 36
   spiritual laws 10

lawyers 22-23, 25, 48, 73, 76, 81-83, 97, 120, 178
   adversity in doctor/patient relationships 23, 82-83

and malpractice 23, 82-83
as healthcare stakeholders 81-83

left-brain thinking 146

Leonard's story 113-119

Letting Go 36, 37, 39, 109-111. *See also* 5 Disciplines of Health Practice

levafloxacin 67

Levaquin 67

life expectancy, U.S. 159

life force 117, 150, 185

Lifelong View 46, 48, 49, 128. *See also* 7 Requirements for Health Practice

light therapy 108

Lipton, Dr. Bruce 172

long term 14, 91
   definition 91

Lyn's story 147-163, 160

M

magnetic resonance imaging: *See* MRI

magnetoencephalography: *See* MEG

malpractice 23, 82-83, 103, 211

mandates 4, 13, 47, 59, 91, 94, 122, 127, 130, 142, 180, 193, 195
   definition 91

Mandela, Nelson 57

map 9-11, 19, 23, 26-27, 100, 123, 197
   the map is not the territory 9

Margaret's story 121

massage 101, 124, 146, 183, 188, 207, 214

McDougall, Dr. John 154

mechanization 13, 90
  definition 13

medical checkup: *See* checkup

medical system 4, 7-9, 20, 23, 24, 32, 33-34, 51, 56, 60, 72, 74-77, 82, 86, 87, 89, 109, 111, 116, 122, 124, 126, 129, 136, 140-143, 149, 160-161, 166-169, 174, 178, 180, 185, 186, 189, 192, 196, 214, 215.
  See also healthcare system
  and technology 86
  disease focus 23
  doctors and 4, 126, 178
  healthcare stakeholders 185
  ICD 20
  new perspective 192
  patients and 24, 60-61, 82, 89, 126, 180
  statistics 74-77

Medicare 22, 66, 74, 75, 85-86, 101, 120, 126, 129, 159, 211
  bankruptcy and 85, 129

medicine 8, 9, 12-13, 17, 22-23, 26, 34, 43-44, 50-52, 56, 61, 63, 66-68, 81-83, 87-89, 90, 91, 99, 100, 107-109, 110, 112, 118, 122-124, 128, 137, 139, 141, 143, 146-155, 157, 162, 166-168, 172, 175-176, 179-180, 182-185, 187-189, 193, 196, 204-215
  alternative 182-184
  conventional medicine 8, 43, 150, 152, 155, 157, 162, 182, 185, 189, 214
  defensive medicine 81-83, 122
  vs. health 196

MEG 99

Melissa's story 63

Menninger, Karl Augustus 50

mentality 63, 124, 129, 151

Merck & Co. 75

metformin 138, 139

Michael's story
  David's friend 64

Michelangelo 149, 151

Millman, Dan 10, 164

mindset 7, 13, 18, 23, 50-51, 76, 91, 129, 132-133, 150

Mindy's story 130-131

Mona Lisa 72-73

MRI 99

Mr. Jones' story 168, 169

multidimensionality 14, 92, 123, 169, 173, 176, 183

myopic perspective 13, 52, 91, 106, 142, 193

Myss, Carolyn 152, 185-186

N

Natasha's brother 66

Natasha's sister 207-214, 217

Natasha's story 204-215

National Center for Complementary and Alternative Medicine 67

National Health Statistics 182, 185

National Institutes of Health 99

231 | THE 7 PRINCIPLES OF HEALTH

National Science Foundation 99

natural laws: *See* laws

naturopathy 94, 124, 146, 153

negative thinking
  power of 19

neurolinguistic programming 19,
99-100

neuroscience 99-101

New Health Model 180

New Health Paradigm 14-16, 19, 91,
102, 142-143, 186, 189, 192-193

new map 19

Newton, Isaac 17

Newtonian physics 13, 17, 90, 123

NLP: *See* neurolinguistic programming

nonjudgment 15, 92
  definition 15

normal 2, 6, 39, 64, 93, 113, 127, 156,
187
  definition 64

nosocomial infection 66-67

Null, Gary 117

nutrition 43, 88, 94, 154, 176, 180, 184,
188

nutrtionists 101, 139, 147, 154-155,
182-183, 188

O

obesity 126, 160

Olson, James 179

opinion 13, 15, 27-28, 38-39, 91-92,
106-109, 155, 182-183

optimal health 5, 9-12, 14, 20, 22,
24-25, 27, 34, 36, 42, 49-50, 58, 65, 70,
73, 92, 94, 102, 105-107, 112, 123, 129,
131, 139, 147, 161-162, 170, 173, 181,
192-193, 207, 215
  alignment with 25
  despite disease labels 27

Osler, Sir William 1, 181

Outside-in, Inside-out 46, 49, 125.
See also 7 Requirements for Health
Practice

P

Pap test 62

paradigm 7, 9, 11, 14-19, 24-27, 32-
35, 43, 49, 56-57, 60-63, 67, 73, 89, 93,
99-100, 106, 108, 123, 133-134, 139-
140, 144, 149, 155, 161, 170, 181, 184,
186, 189, 192, 196, 214.
See also mentality
  definition 7

paradigm shift 7, 16, 18, 56, 61, 161

past-life spiritualist 108

Pastor John's story 43-44, 160

paternalism 13, 91, 94
  definition 13

patient 3-5, 7, 9, 12, 15, 22-23, 26-27,
32, 37-38, 52, 54, 56, 58, 61, 62-66, 68,
72-73, 76, 77, 82-83, 84, 85, 87-89, 99,
101, 106-109, 112, 113, 114, 117-118,
122, 123-127, 129, 133, 135, 154, 157,
160-161, 166-169, 172, 174, 175, 180-
185, 193, 198, 204, 204-214, 216

Patricia's story 64-65, 133-145, 160

232 | THE 7 PRINCIPLES OF HEALTH

Peabody, Dr. Francis W. 190

Penfield, Dr. Wilder 99

penicillin 83-84

Personal Health Mantra 112, 178

PET 99

pharmaceutical companies: *See* drug companies

physicians: *See* doctors

point of view 7-8, 26, 128, 173

polarization 13, 90
  definition 90

positive thinking
  power of 19

positron emission tomography: *See* PET

power to heal 215

practicing medicine vs. practicing health 26

Practicing Now, Daily, and In Moderation 36, 37, 41.
  See also 5 Disciplines of Health Practice

prana 117

prescription drugs 75, 85, 138
  costs 75

principle 10-11, 28-31, 49
  definition 10

Principle 1: Be Present 30-31, 53, 150

Principle 2: Become Aware 31-32, 71, 150

Principle 3: Be Health 33, 98, 151

Principle 4: Reawaken Curiosity 33-

34, 119, 153

Principle 5: Channel Creativity 34-35, 145, 154

Principle 6: Grow and Renew 35, 163

Principle 7: Heal, Change, and Thrive 35-36, 190

profit 45, 52, 78-81, 86, 95, 123, 127, 129, 133, 143, 193, 211
  and disease 52, 86, 95, 143, 193
  and financial imbalance 45

programming 19, 23, 26, 31-32, 93-94, 99-101, 110, 133, 141, 151, 157, 198

Prozac 135

Q

qi 117-118, 185

quantum energy 47, 108

R

reaction 8, 16-19, 21, 44, 76, 104, 109, 127, 133, 136-137
  action vs. 133

Reawaken Curiosity 33, 40, 119, 124, 130, 140, 143, 153, 178, 214.
  See also 7 Principles of Health

Releasing Fear 36, 37, 38
  See also 5 Disciplines of Health Practice

reprogramming 19, 93, 102, 213
  See also programming

Requirement 1: Desire 126

Requirement 2: Commitment 128

Requirement 3: Lifelong View 128

Requirement 4: Self-Accountability 130

Requirement 5: Sequential Steps 131

Requirement 6: Small Steps 132

Requirement 7: Outside-in, Inside-out 133

requirements 11-12, 30-31, 47-51, 125-134, 143
  definition 12

right-brain thinking 146

right here and right now 31, 33, 41, 69, 70, 102, 105, 116, 118, 150, 160, 185.
  See also Be Present

roadmap: *See* map

Robbins, Anthony 99

Role of Stakeholders 77
  doctors 87-89
  drug companies 83-85
  government 85-87
  health insurance companies 77-81
  lawyers 81-83

S

Sagan, Carl 18, 51, 201

scarcity mentality 124

Schweninger M.D., Ernst 71

scripts: *See* programming

Self-Accountability 15, 46, 48, 92, 126, 130.
  See also 7 Requirements for Health Practice
  definition 15

Sequential Steps 46, 49, 131.
  See also 7 Requirements for Health Practice

Serenity Prayer 198

Sharon's story 5-7

Shealy, Dr. Norman 185-186

Sheehy, Gail 135

Siddhartha Gautama 57

Small Steps 46, 49, 125.
  See also 7 Requirements for Health Practice

specialists: *See* doctors

Stopping Judgment 36, 37-38.
  See also 5 Disciplines of Health Practice

strep throat 84

stress 6, 8, 12, 16, 30, 45, 57, 72, 76, 100, 102, 110, 116, 127, 129, 134-135, 150, 170, 172, 183, 186, 204, 207

subconscious 110, 188

T

Tai Chi 176

TCM: *See* Chinese Medicine

teacher: *See* guide

tests 2, 6, 21, 35, 62-63, 82-84, 88, 118, 123, 130, 147-150, 153, 156, 166-169, 184-187

Thoreau, Henry David 25

thought environment 24, 26, 33, 101-105, 151

thoughts 7-8, 16-22, 27-28, 31, 34-

35, 61, 99-106, 110-111, 121, 137, 151-153, 164, 166, 178, 189, 192, 213-215, 216

physical manifestation 19, 189

thought forms 19-20, 33

thrive 35-36, 190, 192, 197-198, 215

Tolle, Eckhart 107, 152

Tracy's story 134-145

Truman, Harry 155

U

unconscious 13, 91, 107, 142, 193

vs. conscious 13, 91, 142, 193

United Health Group 80

urgent care 191, 206-208

U.S. Food and Drug Administration: *See* FDA

V

vancomycin 67

victimization 4-5, 13, 23, 30, 32, 54, 68, 72, 73, 76-77, 80-85, 90, 94, 103, 133, 140-143, 152, 191-193, 215

definition 13

victims: *See* victimization

Vioxx 75

Vitruvian Man 37-41

W

Welch, Jack 131

Wheel of Health Manifestation 157-159, 175, 182, 186

whole 7, 13-14, 16, 17, 23, 65, 72, 89-92, 123, 168, 187, 212

integration of 89

will power 13, 15, 90, 92

World Health Organization 22

Y

Yee, Rodney 212

Your Invitation to Practice Health 56, 69, 81, 95, 111, 117, 136, 144, 146, 162, 164, 170, 176, 194, 196, 201

Made in the USA
San Bernardino, CA
06 April 2013